ADVANCED PRAISE

"*Beyond Powerful* is authentic and hopeful—Lala reminds us of the power already within us"

DR. NICOLE JOHNSON
Miss America 1999

I've often said that I can't regret living with autoimmune disease because that experience helped sculpt who I am. *Beyond Powerful* embraces this positive mindset and takes it to a whole new level, allowing us to appreciate the skills honed through the challenges of chronic illness and, even more importantly, giving us permission to be empowered and improved, yet never defined, by our diseases."

DR. SARAH BALLANTYNE
New York Times bestselling author of *The Paleo Approach*

"She's the perfect prescription of perseverance, authenticity, humor and strength. A must read for anyone looking to become their best selves all while wearing their cape."

NANETTE V.

"I didn't know if I would enjoy reading it because I don't suffer from a chronic illness. I wasn't sure if I would be able to relate. However, the book was filled with so many positive life lessons and stories not only of Lala but other absolutely incredible human beings (some that I had never heard of and that I cannot wait to learn more about!) that I found myself devouring it and applying the concepts to my own life. Lala effortlessly blended the stories of such incredible people with her own life experiences in order to show us all (chronic illness or not) how we can best overcome challenges in order to really realize our self-worth and embrace our opportunities for growth."

AMBER E.

"*Beyond Powerful* is a great read for any superhero out there dealing with chronic illness (or really anyone pursuing huge goals/making major changes in life). It's a fantastic secret weapon to have in your artillery. Read this when you're ready to be inspired to take on the world!"

JENETA H.

"This book is a must read for those struggling with chronic illnesses, those supporting others with chronic illnesses, and even those who have nothing to do with chronic illnesses, but need a reminder that no matter what life throws our way, we have the (super) power to move forward, help others, and achieve our goals—even if sometimes that means stepping aside and taking a deep breath."

MICHAL B.

"Living with chronic illness is no easy feat, but like many other super-humans battling chronic illnesses, Lala has motivated me to push harder to break through the barriers in my life. This book is a priceless resource."

TANEILLE C.

"As a Pediatrician and budding Pediatric Endocrinologist, I knew that I HAD to read this book. I learned so much from it in terms of my interactions with patients and how I can be a better doctor… Whether you have a chronic illness or not… this is a story of coming together, supporting each other, and being proud of what we have! This is a must read."

MARISSA O.

BEYOND
POWERFUL

Your Chronic Illness is
Not Your Kryptonite

LALA JACKSON

NEW YORK

NASHVILLE • MELBOURNE • VANCOUVER

BEYOND POWERFUL

© 2017 Pamela "Lala" Jackson

Published in New York, New York, by Morgan James Publishing in partnership with Difference Press.
www.MorganJamesPublishing.com

The Morgan James Speakers Group can bring authors to your live event. For more information or to book an event visit The Morgan James Speakers Group at www.TheMorganJamesSpeakersGroup.com.

ISBN 978-1-68350-381-1 paperback
ISBN 978-1-68350-382-8 eBook
Library of Congress Control Number:
2016919732

Cover & Interior Design by:
Megan Whitney
Creative Ninja Designs
megan@creativeninjadesigns.com

Editing: Cynthia Kane

Author's Photo:
John Arthur Photography
johnarthurphoto.com

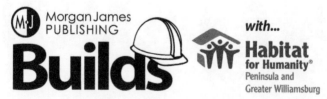

In an effort to support local communities, raise awareness and funds, Morgan James Publishing donates a percentage of all book sales for the life of each book to Habitat for Humanity Peninsula and Greater Williamsburg.

Get involved today! Visit
www.MorganJamesBuilds.com

TABLE OF CONTENTS

ACKNOWLEDGEMENTS

Besides that whole giving me life thing, I can't imagine that much in my life would have gone even remotely well without such constant support from my mom. So first and foremost, thank you mom for being my cheering section, my shoulder to cry on, my biggest advocate, my sounding board, and for playing every possible role in my life. I love you.

Thank you Pete for stepping in when you never had to and making sure that I've had exactly what I needed when everything crumbles. I am lucky to have you around and glad I walked into that West Marine.

Floyd and Nanyo, I know it's weird to basically be three only children, but know that I always carry you both with me. I believe in you deeply.

I have a truly amazing group of friends across the globe, and one of my biggest regrets is that I can't gather all of you in one place so we can be in a weird friend-filled city complete with ridiculously stupid jokes and antics. And also rum punch. There's not enough space in the world to thank you each individually, but you know who you are.

Thank you in particular to La Familia. You ladies and gentlemen have been more of a support than I ever could have imagined, and I am so incredibly lucky to have you all as my father, my brothers and sisters, my aunts and uncles. You! Know!

This writing process was simultaneously crazy and easier than I ever could have imagined it would be, and that is entirely due to my editors Angela Lauria and Cynthia Kane. Thank you for your feedback and your encouragement. To the rest of the team who has tirelessly lent your expertise and support, know that I appreciate you more than you can imagine.

And to you, dear reader, who is going on this journey with me: you are stronger and braver than you even know. Thank you for reading, and please always feel free to reach out to me at lalajackson.com. I hope to see you there!

INTRODUCTION
HOW DID I GET HERE?

On Thanksgiving Day when I was ten years old, I ended up in the intensive care unit of Seattle Children's Hospital. That September I had started sixth grade at a new, prestigious college prep school and despite being generally known as a precocious learner and voracious reader, my teachers doubted if it was the place for me – I was constantly lethargic and seemed disinterested in my work.

In the months leading up to the holidays, I had lost nearly thirty pounds on a 5'4" frame that didn't have the weight to lose; multiple doctors told my mom I was doing it on purpose to somehow better fit in with my new peers. I have flashes of memories from that time – trying and failing to eat a single scrambled egg but downing 2-liters of Sprite daily. Barely being able to walk up the hill to my school's gym. Lots of lying around in bed. A very frustrated mom who was trying to pack up the family home so we could move over the holiday weekend.

At about four o'clock in the morning on Thanksgiving day, my mom tried, unsuccessfully, to wake me up. One of her co-worker's kids had just been put into the hospital for bacterial meningitis, never to be the same jovial nine-year-old again, and she was terrified that I was about to go down the same path. My family carried me to our old Jeep Cherokee and tried to put me in the back seat, but I couldn't sit up on my own. My entire body hurt. So they put me in the way back, the place I always begged to sit but wasn't allowed to because of the lack of seatbelts, and we pelted down the highway toward the closest hospital, Overlake Medical Center.

Moments after I was carried into the emergency room, a nurse came over to check on me. She smelled my sweet breath, which should have been a dead giveaway to all the doctors who said these health issues were my own doing. She instantly diagnosed me with the autoimmune disease type one diabetes (T1D).

After being somewhat stabilized in the emergency room, I was put into an ambulance and taken to Seattle Children's Hospital, where I spent two days in the intensive care unit, then another two as an inpatient, learning what had happened to my body and how to check my blood sugar levels and give myself insulin shots. It was my new normal and one that would never go away. There was no cure. They didn't know what caused the disease. I had no family history. Possible future complications included kidney failure, loss of eyesight, amputation, and premature death.

Sitting in the patient education room, the clinical diabetes educator tried to teach me how to give myself shots with syringes. I practiced on an orange first. Then on my teddy bear. When my next step was to practice on my mom, to give her a shot of saline, I completely broke down. I could do everything else. I could prick my fingers. I could learn to count carbohydrates. I could skip regular soda. At ten, when everything was an adventure, I could adjust to this new life. But I could not hurt my mom, and I could not hurt myself. The nurses tried to explain that this was the only way to keep myself alive and healthy, but all I saw was my purposely shoving a sharp object under my skin and it broke me.

I eventually learned because I had to, but for the first year my mom still gave me my shots. When she was out of town, we taught my older brother how. Gadgets and technology have since made my life easier, but to this day, if my routine changes, if I have to use a new type of needle, if my insulin pump infusion sets, which work like mini-IVs, change design, you will find me in a puddle of tears, trying to give myself a pep talk that it's not going to be so bad. It's never the pain – the needles don't hurt that much. But they do leave little bruises and scars, little reminders that this is never going away, little visual cues that at the end of the day, shoving these needles into my stomach, backside, thighs, and arms – it isn't normal.

In that first year, my doctor sent me to a psychiatrist about this fear of needles. He was worried that it was going to prevent my ability to take care of myself. After an hour in the psychiatrist's office, she and I agreed – I would only need to come back if I suddenly developed a love for needles. At that point, she'd be worried.

My fear has never kept me from giving myself the medicine I need to live, but I'm still scared of needles. As a grown adult who has been through far worse things (dammit), I have a tendency to pass out when I have to get blood drawn. When I had to have surgery a few years ago on a badly broken ankle, it wasn't the surgery I was scared of. It was the needles that had to be shoved into my knee to numb the nerves traveling down my leg. But needles are and will always be a part of my everyday existence. I remain scared of them. I use them anyway.

And that got me thinking – how much in my life has probably been affected by that every day practice of bravery? How many other situations have there been where I was scared of the THING but I did the THING anyway, because that was what I was in the practice of doing? I was a blunt, headstrong little kid, but as I've grown up, how much has my disease taught me to barrel ahead even more so than I ever could have done without it?

As I was starting to formulate what this book would be, I knew that the element of courage was important to me – one that I think far more of us possess than we give ourselves credit for. It was my plan to keep this research on bravery restricted to the world of women being kickass leaders, and how our bravery is such an important element in that. It is what allows us to go after the new opportunities, make the speech even though we're scared of speaking in front of crowds, chase the promotion even though it's an entirely new playing field, start the business without any guarantee it's going to work. Do it all while juggling a million other things, a million other expectations, and somehow coming out on the other side with grace and a usually intact sense of humor.

And, as it goes, as I delved into this topic further, I was getting more and more sick. My immune system was on the fritz. I was exhausted. My body was hurting. I was constantly in a fog. I couldn't formulate the thoughts I wanted. And I realized I was absolutely full of it.

I was trying to create this rallying cry around being our most courageous selves while being leaders in everything we pursued without addressing the very real thing I was dealing with at the time – being truly sick. My immune system was dive-bombing and I was trying to talk about being brave enough to be an empowered boss babe. I wasn't addressing what was actually going on with me, or what goes on with so many of us overachieving women who are also battling this constant force of not being well.

And how do you address that? How do you come to terms with the fact that you're trying to get stuff done, but you feel like hell? That you feel like a slacker because your body is holding you back from a goal? That you feel like your sickness is betraying what you know you can accomplish?

The truth is, as far I can tell, these thoughts always come up. I cannot think of a single person I know who lives with chronic disease and hasn't dive-bombed into a place of feeling like a burden, feeling like they're never going to get better, feeling hopeless and fragile, feeling like there's nothing they can do to help themselves. We don't always admit to these thoughts – we're not the types to give in to them. But they float through sometimes. They tend to be unwelcome visitors in the middle of the night as we're lying on the bathroom floor because the tile is cool against our aching bodies. They pop up when we're in the doctor's office, again, because they can't figure out what's wrong this time. They visit us a few hours after we've eaten something that we realized, far too late, is going to make the next few days a nauseated hell.

Our friends and well-meaning family will remind us that we're fighters, that we're stronger than this, that it's going to get better. But is it? These are things with our health that aren't going to just disappear, so how do we learn to exist with them, day in, day out? How do we learn to make peace with them? To chase the things anyway, knowing that there might be days when we have no other choice than to take a time out?

As I've gotten the incredible chance to talk to more and more women dealing with these health hurdles on a daily basis (want to join in? *Amazing conversations happen over in our Facebook community. Just search for my page HeyLalaJackson),* I've learned that we're far stronger than we realize. And maybe, just maybe, these diseases we deal with helped make us so.

I know, I know, screw this disease. It hasn't helped you one bit. I get it. I do.

When I was first diagnosed with T1D, days out of the intensive care unit, my pediatric endocrinologist, Dr. Gad Kletter, insisted that I go on my scheduled backcountry snowshoeing trip. My school, in its very Pacific Northwest way, had an outdoor education requirement and this trip was part of my yearly credits. I can only imagine the panic this had to have sent my mom into. Sending her newly diagnosed ten year old daughter who absolutely did not know how to take care of herself yet into the woods with no cell phone service and no roads to do intense exercise which could easily drop her blood sugar and send her into a seizure. I'm not sure I would have let me go had I been in her position. But let me go she did.

I was fine. Nothing bad happened. I had a blast, I rolled around in the snow with my classmates, and I was taught from very early on that I could do absolutely anything I wanted to do despite my disease. It may cause interruptions, but it would never hold me back. It was exactly what Dr. Kletter had wanted me to learn.

It was an approach I always took. Can I fly halfway across the world to go on a three week trip around Europe? Sure! Can I camp on a remote island, only accessible by boat, in the Sea of Cortez for a week? Why not! Can I pursue a goal of being an Olympic rower? Absolutely (or until I injured my wrist from completely non-diabetes related issues)! Can I go to college 6,000 miles away from home in a state in which I have never touched foot? Great idea!

It wasn't until my last year at the University of Miami, where I attended five years of undergrad (I was an overzealous student leader who tended to put my organizational involvement ahead of my classwork. Oops. Expensive oops.), that someone finally gave me a big fat "no" on the grounds of my disease.

After going through nine months of clearance for the Peace Corps to work in health promotion, I was denied medical clearance because of my health. The particularly frustrating thing was that I knew people with T1D who served in the Peace Corps. I've known more since. I tried to fight the decision, but it turns out that whoever reviews your file gets final say. It was the luck of the draw.

I was devastated. It was the first time in my life that I couldn't do something because of my disease, and I didn't even get to make the choice. I know now that that's when I started shrinking myself. I had been so passionate about working in health promotion and education, particularly for people who lived with chronic disease like I did. But I stopped chasing it. I didn't want anything to do with it anymore. I accepted a business internship that I didn't really care about and moved to a city that I never felt drawn to. I accepted a full time job there. I moved further and further into the suburbs. Further and further into safe territory. I stopped living boldly. I stopped being creative. I got really angry with myself and my disease. I became incredibly harsh on myself. It resulted in a six-year decline of my health, in excessive weight gain, in another autoimmune crash. I was completely out of alignment and I had let my disease start running my life. And of course I didn't realize it at the time.

With that one decision made for me, I allowed every decision afterward to be affected too. I was letting my sickness limit me without realizing that that's what I had done.

Hindsight is a hell of a thing. In our Facebook community, I was able to have a chat with a woman named Julia, who, while living and dealing with chronic disease, had been advised to do the same thing by her medical care team. "Take it easy, maybe you don't need to be in school right now, maybe you don't need to be in that relationship right now, maybe you should avoid contact with your family, we wouldn't want you to stress yourself further."

I don't know Julia personally but I love her because she told her care team to shove it. As she said on our page, she recognized that "stress isn't always from doing something; sometimes it's [from] not doing it enough." She stayed in school. She found funding aid to help her keep studying and get the support she needed. She got married to her boyfriend. She maintains contact with her family. Her disease isn't going anywhere, but she chose to truly live fully instead of sitting back and letting her sickness run the show.

What are we missing out on when we let our sicknesses limit us? It did nothing for me except slowly kill off my passion for my own life. I let myself be talked into taking the safer route rather than living to the full extent of my abilities, and it was a long and painful road to get back to a place where I even recognized myself again.

As that fog has lifted, I've realized something so important. We are the overachievers, the dreamers, the doers, so what does it do for us to limit ourselves? Yes, we will always live with our diseases, but they don't get to choose our path. Only we do.

It is absolutely possible to be both chronically ill and achieve amazing things. Our sicknesses have made us learn how to prioritize, delegate, and be assertive; all things that people pay thousands upon thousands of dollars to master in leadership development courses. We can translate those skills into our goals, and we can make this work FOR us instead of against us. Our diseases may make every step of the way harder, they interrupt us from time to time, but they're not stopping us from doing great things.

So allow me to present a different option besides letting our diseases run our lives, the option of embracing this odd little dichotomy of ours. Because I think living with our particular chronic disease soups have given us super powers.

There's a certain set of skills that comes with having always had to be our own advocates. Sticking up for ourselves and telling a highly educated doctor who's a rock-star in her field that we think she doesn't have something right. Knowing that it's a rough day but we're going to get our project done anyway. Learning to love ourselves, with our many imperfections. Saying 'no' when we need to take care of ourselves and trusting that the right opportunity isn't going to skip over us just because we need to prioritize self-care. Taking advantage of the days when we feel well and going on adventures. Knowing when it's time to ask for help. Being courageous enough to chase a near-impossible goal. Being courageous enough to take time off to take care of ourselves.

Call me crazy, but I don't know many people who have the gift of perfect health who know how to do each of these things. I think they are things that can come only when we're faced with this particular set of adversities.

Do we feel strong enough to practice each of these every day? Nope. But are we capable? More than. Is that a surprise? Well, love, you're already great, and you didn't even know it. You are already a leader, there are already people who look up to you for everything you tackle, and even though you have days when you feel like absolute crap, you are a beacon for others fighting through the same.

And that's what I encourage you to take away from this book. That you are powerful. You are strong. I'm here to tell you how.

In the coming chapters, I am going to show you how to embrace these different sides of yourself. Yes, you live with sickness. But you are also a powerhouse. You are capable of reaching every goal you set for yourself. This isn't just some pie-in-the-sky thing. By living with chronic disease, you have already learned the skills to be great. You just didn't acquire them in the most traditional of ways.

Now, let's take a minute to acknowledge a few things. One, every single person reading this book is going to be walking a different path of health. I get that. But no matter if you are bed-bound or live with a completely invisible illness that allows you to navigate the world with relative normality most of the time, by merely picking up this book to read it, I know that you are someone who is capable of great things. Why? Because you want to be. The will to be great is all you need to be great, because your will is your vision, and with your vision, you can make anything happen.

Two, only you get to set your definition of over-achieving. Whatever you want to bring to the world, it is enough. And however you choose to do it, it is enough. If we all lived within the same confines of what being a go-getter should be, we would live in an incredibly boring world. Being a powerhouse in your own right does not have to mean running a massive company, starting a successful tech business, or being anyone else's vision of high-achieving. Being a go-getter just means bringing what you want to the world and not allowing anything to limit you. You make your own rules here.

This book exists to help you navigate that weird space of being that overachieving person who lives with something that wipes you out sometimes. I'm here to say that it's okay. That you might get wiped out again and again, but you will also get up again and again. Because you already know how. You're in the practice of it.

LET'S TALK SCIENCE & STATS

I'm willing to bet that if you're reading this book, you probably identify as a woman (if not, hello to one of my estimated five male readers!). And you're probably the type to push yourself through new goals, be they academic, artistic, business, or personal. No matter what it is, you have a tendency to GO for it. You sometimes realize you just took on WAY more than you know how to handle, but you always figure it out. The really cool thing? That's not uncommon for women. We've always been powerhouses, but advances over the last few decades, led by courageous women opening the doors before us, have given us the opportunity to achieve in ways we never before imagined.

Before we get into the nitty-gritty, I want to take a moment to say two key things. One, BRA-flippin'-VO. I'm proud of us. I'm proud of all we continue to chase, all the goals we set, and how much we support each other. I think being part of a tribe of women who aren't afraid to strive high and give each other high-fives and legs up on the way to the top is a magical thing. Two, the upcoming statistics are general to American women, and do not account for differences in social, racial, or economic classes, nor for differences faced by women in other parts of the world. They do not account for the specific set of burdens certain groups of women face and for that I am sorry. I knew in writing this book that I could go on for hundreds of pages to include disparities and differences from country to country, which are so important to acknowledge when we're talking about all that women have accomplished and all that we still face. Alas, it's information that I could not do justice here. So the upcoming information is based on all American women as a general, broad-stroke category. Now let's get into it.

In 1970, 34 percent of women in the workforce were high school drop outs (per the US Department of Labor Bureau of Labor Statistics (BLS)). More than a third! Since then, across the board, not only are women able to stay in school at a significantly higher rate (in 2015, just eight percent of women in the workforce had dropped out of high school), but we are going on to earn degrees at a higher rate than men. As reported by the Washington Post in 2014, "Women today get the majority of college degrees in America. It doesn't matter what kind – associate's, bachelor's, master's, or doctoral – women beat men in all the categories. In the 2009-2010 academic year, women earned 57.4 percent of all bachelor's degrees." The only exception to this rule, as reported by the Harvard Business Review, is MBAs, where women earn nearly 40 percent of degrees. Within the labor force, BLS reports that 40 percent of working women, ages 25 to 64, have college degrees, versus just 11.2 percent of working women who had a post-secondary degree in 1970.

With higher education, we are contributing financially and becoming our families' breadwinners at a higher rate. As noted by the BLS, less than one-third of women worked outside of the home immediately following World War II, whereas 60 percent worked outside of the home in 1999. The bureau also reported that in 1987, in households where both partners worked, just 17.8 percent of women earned more than their husbands. By 2010, that number had increased to 28.2 percent. That of course doesn't take into account earnings from families outside of husband-wife reporting, which are becoming more and more common.

So we're becoming more highly educated, we're starting to earn more, and guess what else? We're becoming bosses at a higher and higher rate. Per Entrepreneur.com, women own 10.6 million businesses in the United States and employ 19.1 million workers, which is one in every seven employees. We're paying $492 billion in salaries. I haven't done the math there, but that is an estimated hell of a lot of lives we're supporting. Our businesses account for $2.5 trillion in sales.

In traditional companies, women account for 40 percent of managers. While we are far from equally represented, 16 percent of the c-suite of Fortune 500 companies are now comprised of women, and companies whose c-suites are at least 30 percent women show a higher profit than companies with less or without (as reported by the Harvard Business Review). We still need to keep fighting for further representation; clearly it would benefit not only women but also American business as a whole. But we are moving in the right direction (however slowly).

Are we earning the same money for the same work? Nope. As reported in the American Community Survey, as of 2014, women made 79 cents for every dollar a man earned for the same work. The gender pay gap increases with age and is worse for women of color, mothers, and women who live in certain states (generally women who live in the Deep South and the Midwest see the largest gap – shoutout to Washington D.C., New York, and Hawaii with 90 cents, 87 cents, and 86 cents earned to the dollar, respectively – you get to claim the 'not as awful' award). On our current track, the gender pay gap will not close for another 100 years or more. Per the American Association of University Women, while higher education helps, there is statistically no level of education that can be attained to close the gap completely.

But I'm willing to bet that the readers of this book can take that particular issue on should they feel so inclined. Because, as I'll explain further in our remaining chapters, I think we have a particular set of skills. Skills that we've acquired over a very long life of living with chronic disease. Skills that I think make us superheroes who aren't afraid to back down from a worthy fight. Yes, that was a "Taken" reference. And yes, I think you all can make it happen.

Alongside all of this increasingly good news about women being generally awesome human beings in the world of getting things done, we're unfortunately also being faced with a very sad, very scary truth. We are getting sicker. Have you seen the movie "Wall-E"? Where humans have gotten so lazy that our entire existence is in recliner chairs with screens in front of us and readily available food? That's part of it – the movie wasn't far off. But in addition to health issues related to increasing rates of obesity and other lifestyle related factors, rates of autoimmune and otherwise non-preventable diseases are also increasing.

The National Institutes of Health (NIH) estimates that up to 23.5 million Americans suffer from autoimmune disease and that the prevalence is rising. Other organizations, such as the American Autoimmune Related Disease Association (AARDA), put that number at closer to 50 million, stating that the NIH numbers only include a limited breadth of diseases and do not encompass full statistics. Over the past few decades, researchers at AARDA have identified 80 to 100 different autoimmune diseases and have found possible autoimmune ties to an additional 40 diseases. The fun part? It's estimated that of all Americans living with autoimmune disease, more than 75 percent of them are women. Wonderful.

Chronic diseases come in every variety imaginable - they affect all systems and are not always recognized by the medical community, since they come in so many different forms and present in so many different ways. Autoimmune diseases in particular happen when the body's immune system has a snafu and decides that it's time to kill off or impair a vital part of the body's normal function. I posit that my immune system, which managed to kill off the part of my pancreas that creates vital hormones to keep me alive, now suffers from self-confidence issues. I've always pictured a nerdy little blob with glasses slamming his head against the wall whenever he realizes he's let yet another infection go by. Thank you, Pixar and Disney for creating the "Inside Out" characters in the exact replica of what I always thought my off-beat immune system looked and acted like.

In Donna Jackson Nakazawa's 2009 book, *The Autoimmune Epidemic*, she explores possible reasons why autoimmune diseases are on such a sharp rise. As stated in the book's foreword written by Douglas Kerr, M.D., Ph. D., autoimmune diseases are, in some cases, three times more prevalent than they were just a few decades ago. One in twelve Americans, and one in nine American women will develop at least one autoimmune condition at some point in our lifetime.

While scientists and doctors are not in agreement about what is causing this to happen, they can agree on one thing - something is clearly wrong. The increased rates of disease are not due to an increase in ability to diagnose them, but truly due to the crashing of our immune systems. Theories range from a general overtaxing of our systems due to increased toxins we are exposed to on a daily basis, to us no longer being exposed to enough naturally-occurring germs and bacteria to develop our immune systems correctly. The 'cleanliness is next to godliness' philosophy spread widely in response to the types of infectious diseases that swept through populations may have kept certain humans from contracting a plague, but it also kept us away from the very things that helped our immune systems stay balanced.

In Moises Velasquez-Manoff's book *An Epidemic of Absence*, he explores how autoimmune diseases and allergies could be due to a misfiring immune system, no longer knowing how to function correctly in the absence of a once carefully balanced internal ecosystem that actually specifically evolved to coexist with parasites. In the absence of these parasites, the immune system overreacts to everything else, creating a warlike internal state.

Recent research from JDRF, the leading organization for type 1 diabetes (T1D) research, is looking into the microbiome of the gut and how it differs for people who are diagnosed with T1D in comparison to people without. In I-am-somehow-not-at-all-surprised news, researchers found that the healthy flora significantly decreases in the gut the year before diagnosis, and they don't yet know why.

Unfortunately, women also bear the brunt when it comes to mental illness, another major player in the chronic disease arena. According to the World Health Organization (WHO), one in three people, predominately women, have experienced depression or anxiety. Depression is twice as common in women (12 percent of American women have experienced depression, versus six percent of American men), and is suspected to be more persistent in women than in men.

The tie between other chronic illnesses and mental illness is strong – those who live with physical chronic diseases are far more likely to also deal with mental illness, and it is not purely due to the stress the physical condition creates. When your system is not in balance, everything goes hay-wire. And when the majority of serotonin, the chemical in your body that acts as a mood stabilizer, among other things, is made in the gut and used throughout your body, it is absolutely zero surprise that diseases affecting the rest of your system would affect your mental health as well, and vice versa.

Of course there are a myriad of other chronic illnesses not caused by lifestyle, for which there is no prevention and no cure. And yet we live with them. Day in, day out. And honestly, it's scary sometimes. It just is what it is. How do we not let fear take over and paralyze us?

In the same way, when we're chasing a giant goal – one that we're not entirely sure we have the know-how or ability to accomplish – how do we not let our own fear get in the way before we even have the chance to try?

Eleanor Roosevelt, who forever changed the role of the American President's First Lady, once said, "you gain strength, courage, and confidence by every experience in which you really stop and look fear in the face. You must do the thing which you think you cannot do."

Not only solid advice from a solid lady, but scientifically sound. Rod Hairston, a speaker, coach, and author who specializes in developing human potential, often speaks on the science of fear. At a conference where he presented in 2015, I learned that when humans are faced with an unknown situation, our bodies are designed to use our own fear as a way to protect us from a potentially harmful situation. The problem? Our body and biological system responds in the same exact way, no matter if the situation you happen to be facing at the time is being precariously close to falling over the edge of a cliff, or about to go on a date with the kindest human on the planet. Either way, the body is screaming "HEY! WE DON'T KNOW WHAT'S GOING ON HERE!" and is sincerely trying to help us out by giving the cues of sweaty palms, racing heart, and shaking limbs. To the human brain and body, fear is fear. It's a protective mechanism. The brain fears what it does not yet know.

It's helpful in the situations where we may actually be getting into something dangerous – learning to trust our gut is a massive skill. But what about the times when our body is trying to protect us from something that could actually really benefit us? How do we get past that gnawing feeling in our gut to do something great? By doing it. By breaking the pattern the fear is creating.

Dr. Joe Dispenza is a world renowned author and speaker who I had the great luck to see speak in 2016. He specializes in neuroscience and quantum physics, particularly around how the brain and its neural pathways function and can be rewired based on thoughts and experiences. What are neural pathways? Not to have already referenced the Pixar/Disney movie "Inside Out" twice in the matter of a few pages (it's a great movie, okay?), but they explained it perfectly. Based on past experiences, our brain creates memories. When a memory is particularly impactful, it becomes a part of who we are. Without even being able to remember what the memory is, it creates our personality. If we have a warehouse full of happy, joyous memories, we tend to be happy, joyous people. If we have a particularly negative or traumatic experience, that becomes a part of our personality as well. The pathway has been created. The good thing is, the pathway can also be rewired. How? By noticing it exists.

We've talked about how I have a fear of needles. About how, even now, two decades into using them on a daily basis, I still get all weepy and lightheaded when I have to deal with them in any unplanned situation. As I write this book, over the past few weeks I have gotten a variety of blood tests done as doctors are trying to figure out some new issues I am having with intense pain and inflammation (chronic illness life, amiright?).

In my first doctor's visit, I knew I was probably going to have to have a few vials of blood taken. I had prepared for it — I drank a lot of water in the day and morning before. I did breathing exercises. I envisioned feeling fine while and after the blood was taken. I sent happy thoughts to the vein in the top of my left hand which remains the only vein that ever successfully gives blood (I get that that's extremely woo-woo, but I'm to the point in my life where I'm going to go ahead and shrug at you and say "whatever works!").

In another doctor's appointment a week later, they ordered another round of tests. I had not expected this. I froze up as soon as my endocrinologist said, "let's run some tests and see what's going on here." I felt tears start to gather behind my eyes. I tried to breathe through it. I warned the phlebotomist that I tend to get a little woozy. Full disclosure — the only time in my adult life I allowed a lab to take more than three vials of blood at a time, I passed out and threw up on myself. Lovely, right? I looked at my still-bruised left hand hoping my single, trusty vein would hold up. I thought about the water I should have been drinking. My palms got sweaty. Halfway through the second vial, I started to get lightheaded. I hadn't been prepared, I hadn't thought about creating a positive experience, so that fear pathway took over.

Not to completely psychoanalyze myself, but for the purposes of this book, I started exploring why I have this massive fear neural pathway built up around needles. Somehow I had never really taken the time to think this through before, but as I sat down to write, I started laughing because it was so obvious. When I was diagnosed with T1D, I was severely dehydrated and about to slip into a coma from months of living with an undiagnosed and therefore untreated disease. My body was barely functioning as it had had no way to turn my food into fuel for months. The basic systems to keep me alive were slowly shutting down from lack of energy. Luckily, I was not conscious for this process, but my mom has told me that as the nurses were trying to find a vein in which to put an IV for fluids and insulin, they tried my arms, my hands, my feet, my legs, all unsuccessfully. They left marks all over my body trying to frantically find a way to deliver me the medicines and fluids needed to make sure I didn't slip into a permanent coma or die. When I woke up in the ICU, unsure of where I was, vaguely aware of a soft blue blinking light in the room, my neck had an intense aching feeling on one side. I tried to start massaging the pain away, but when I put my hand to my neck, there were tubes sticking out of it. Unable to place an IV anywhere else, they had placed one in one of my jugular veins. Getting that IV removed a day later as I was transferred out of the ICU is in my top five most painful experiences.

Memories of a painful thing are hard to relive. We are wired, at a biological level, to avoid that kind of pain. Every time I am now faced with a needle, my brain and my body are trying to protect me from ever going through that again. The only way I can break that association down is to acknowledge it, and coax my brain and body along like a tiny child. "It's okay, it's not going to hurt you again. Look! That wasn't so bad! We're fine, shhhhhh, we're fine."

It's weird. It's weird to have to be our own coaches through these fear-based processes, but we must. As our body and brains try to protect us, we have to acknowledge what's going on to break that pattern of association.

The fear is the same, whether you're dealing with a massive health meltdown, or sitting at your desk until the wee hours of the morning in a cold sweat, wondering how on earth you're going to reach a goal you set for yourself. The fear kicks in, the self-doubt, but it's important to recognize that it's coming from a place that your body only thinks it knows.

If the last time you aimed for a massive goal and you didn't make it, your body will assume that that's what now is going to happen every time. It's going to try to protect you from going through pain again, whether the pain is physical or mental. The only way to break through the fear barrier is to recognize it, then run straight through it. Otherwise, you're just reinforcing what your body and brain thinks it knows – that this thing you're doing will only end badly, so let's not go there. It's up to you to train yourself through that, to help your own mind recognize that you can, in fact, reach this new goal. That there's nothing to be protected from. Once you create that pattern, over and over again, your body will get used to you going there, and will no longer react with that cold sweat fear.

The odd thing is, this is a strictly human problem. Consider the fight or flight instinct, which is also based around deeply ingrained neural pathways. All animals have a fight or flight instinct, humans included. There's a key difference, though, that I learned in an analogy shared by Dr. Dispenza.

When an animal in the wild is being preyed upon, they flee or they fight. This is an ingrained response based purely on survival. When the running or the fighting is done and they've come out on the other side, all of the adrenaline, hormones, and concern about what just happened goes away. They go on about whatever it was they were trying to do in the first place. It's life, and it goes on. They will learn to become more cautious about situations that could bring them true danger, but the caution won't be emotion-based.

When a human feels like they're in a 'preyed upon' situation (and this could be anything from actually being assaulted, just running into someone they've decided they don't like for whatever reason, or any other number of situations), they "flee" or they "fight" (leave the situation, stay and argue, stay and stew in their feelings, shoot the side-eye with a vengeance, whatever else), and then they stay thinking about the thing for however long they allow themselves to. Hours. Weeks. Months. Years. Those stress hormones, the adrenaline, the panic - they stay in our system for as long as we allow them to. Those neural pathways are created not just once, but again, and again, and again, for however long we allow the process to go on. If we allow them to stay for one day, it's just a thing that happened that we can get over. If we allow them to stay for days or weeks, it's a mood that we can snap out of. But when we allow ourselves to dwell for months or years, this becomes a part of our personality. And it is truly difficult to get rid of.

Evolution helped us out by creating these pathways - creating basic human reactions to stimuli so that, instead of staying in a bad situation to slowly assess what's going on, we have the automatic reaction to protect ourselves. In many situations, it saves our lives, keeps us from getting hurt, or at least keeps us from making the same stupid mistake over and over again. But by making us thinking individuals, it also gifted us with the opportunity to learn to let that stuff go, or not. The choice is ours.

The trick is to make sure you're not letting your brain, or fear, keep you in a place that no longer serves you. That place could be related to your health, your business, or whatever else.

It is perfectly reasonable to acknowledge a fear. To recognize why it's happening. To even thank your mind and body for trying to protect you by making it show up. But there comes a time when you have to tell it to go away, that it can go sit in the corner, that it has no place here. That you're busy, so don't interrupt. Please and thank you.

What's really cool, I think, is that by living with something that makes you confront fear so consistently, and with so much power, you've probably already been doing this quite often even if you weren't recognizing the mechanics or biology behind it. Living with any kind of chronic health issue requires a great deal of courage and brings about a particular set of superpowers – yes, superpowers – that can only be gained through life with such a persistent weight on our shoulders.

SUPERPOWER #1
VOICE

My mom is one of the kindest humans I know. In my entire lifetime, we've gotten in four arguments – two about my health, one about dating, and one about figuring out what I was going to do after I got my denial letter from the Peace Corps. It had sent me on a several months-long downward spiral during which I wanted to do literally nothing else with my life. In each, she never yelled. She does the far scarier thing of getting really quiet and saying she's disappointed. Mom kung fu.

When I was getting into my later teenage years and starting to navigate the world of doctors, insurance, and pharmacies on my own, I would often have to tap mom into the game once I felt like I had exhausted my options. Inevitably, the next time I would go to the pharmacy to pick up the medicine they were previously showing as not covered by insurance and therefore $500+ for the month, I would say my name and they would respond with, "RIGHT! Right. Yes, we have it right here. So sorry. So sorry about that. Nope, just $20. So sorry," and I would get SUPER curious about what the hell happened when my mom called.

I found out one day in high school back home in Honolulu. My school was on a block system, so we only had three classes a day for two hours each. Our senior year, every now and then we'd get a block free. If it was the first block or the last block, we could come late or leave early, but if it was the middle block, we weren't supposed to leave campus. It just so happened that on one of these occasions when I had a middle block, I needed to run to the store to get batteries for my insulin pump, which was about to die. As soon as I mentioned this to the front office staff, they let me leave without another question asked. When I got back to the office to check in, I joked around about having gone on a joy ride and they didn't question me. A 17-year-old with a car on a school day allowed to leave for the first time and they were acting like they trusted me entirely – something was not right. I pressed a bit more to try to figure out why they let me go.

"Girl, we are on STRICT instructions to let you do what you need for your diabetes."

"What? From who?"

"Your mom. She was very clear. VERY clear. She's tough, yea?"

I laughed, but in a way it's true – as kind as she is, my mom is my fierce protector and will not accept no as an answer when that no is interfering with my well-being. It's not fierce protector in a screaming, yelling way. It is always a firm, well-reasoned, "you WILL help us with this" statement. It becomes impossible to say no to her.

She once wrote a 100-page scientifically-researched document and sent a copy to my insurance company, my medical provider, my medical technology company, and the state's insurance commissioner, with whom she had made friends, to get a new piece of blood sugar monitoring technology covered by my insurance. She is tireless. And it taught me something key – in many cases, if you get creative, are willing to work, know your stuff, and refuse to accept no as an answer, you can usually get to a yes. I think that's a really special thing we get to learn through the process of navigating life with a chronic disease.

Creators, founders, authors, CEOs – they all have to wade through a sea of negative answers before they get to a yes. The key is that they keep going. In all of those situations, they could decide to give up, they could decide to accept the no. We know about people like Steve Jobs, Oprah Winfrey, the Wright brothers, Albert Einstein, Fred Astaire, Bill Gates, Lucille Ball, Michael Jordan, and J.K. Rowling because they failed first but kept going. I could fill books with a list of names of people who had to be their own advocates when no one else believed they deserved what they were asking for – a break, a job, a spot on a team, a publishing deal. But there's something key here – every single one of these people had the option to throw in the towel. It is only through sheer grit and determination that they decided not to, that they decided to keep going.

When it is your life on the line, your health, your well-being, you don't have the option to give up. You must be your own advocate. It's tiring. It makes you want to scream and cry and throw your shoe at the people who just aren't getting the fact that you truly do need what you're asking for. But in a way, isn't that special? You can navigate medical bureaucracy like a silent ninja (or a bullish pro-wrestler, when need be), always getting to your end goal, whatever that end goal is. Think of how much else that can be applied to.

You have learned to not accept no as an answer because you had to learn. You have the resilience of which others dream. I know it doesn't always feel like it, but think about this - if you can get the physician's assistant to give you sample medication because you know you can't afford the cost of your new prescription right now, you can convince your business idol to look at your business proposal. If you can write a compelling enough letter to the trial administrators to get them to consider you for a limited-spot clinical trial, you can write a compelling enough introduction to get that editor to consider your book idea. If you can run the science experiment that is your body, day in, day out, considering all of the data and carefully measuring it against your own historical data to see how a new nutrition and exercise routine is affecting your health, you can write the code for that iPhone app you've been mulling over.

By living with this disease, you have learned how to be your own advocate with your doctors, nurses, teachers, school administrators, boss, advisors, parents, and friends. You know how to stick up for yourself. You know what you need and what you're capable of. When that perfect storm of being sure about what you know and being willing to keep fighting happens, you can often get to the yes you require.

Over the past decade, the technology used to care for T1D has drastically improved. The most game-changing piece of equipment has been the continuous glucose monitor, generally known as a CGM, which is a little sensor that sits right under your skin and takes a blood sugar level reading every five minutes. It provides an almost overwhelming amount of data, but is the biggest key to having the insight needed to help make my body function as close to a non-diabetic's as possible. For a very long time, this system was cost-prohibitive for me and it continues to be for a lot of people, but I was finally able to pursue getting it in April of 2016 with new insurance that would cover it at 100 percent. I cried when I found that out. Big tears, ugly face cried. My blood sugar levels had never acted as they were "supposed" to and I was often listed as "non-compliant" by my medical teams, despite my trying incredibly hard to get my blood sugar levels in a better range. Having this tool would be life-changing for me. It was a big deal.

I called the medical technology company, all my insurance information in hand and ready to go, the day I qualified for coverage. A few days later, they told me they were ready to ship out my order for the low, low price of $864. I explained to them that my insurance covered the system at 100 percent and to please run everything through again.

Over the course of the next two months, I had almost daily communication with my insurance company, the medical technology company, and my work's benefits manager. The medical technology company was completely over me – they thought I was not only wrong about my insurance coverage, but I got the impression they thought I was also irritating and pushy. I made a massive point of being as pleasant as possible to everyone involved even though I knew that someone was messing up. I ended up having to track down the codes needed to run everything through correctly and acting as a liaison between the companies, translating what forms needed to be filled out and by whom, tracking conversations that should have been tracked in their systems, and reiterating what ICD-10 and CPT codes were needed to make everything go through correctly. In June, when everything finally went through the system, the medical technology company representative seemed genuinely surprised that I was right about all of the coverage after all. I've found that surprise is usually the reaction to anyone actually knowing their stuff. Within the chronic disease-having population, I really don't think it's that rare. We have to know it.

If I hadn't fought for so long and chosen to inform myself about every step of the process, I never would have gotten this tool that has now drastically changed how I can take care of myself. If I had gotten embarrassed about calling so much, if I had assumed that maybe I was wrong, if I hadn't been so persistent, I either would not have gotten the needed tool, or I would have been almost a thousand dollars out of pocket, plus the extra few hundred dollars I'd need every month to keep my supplies stocked.

I cried more than a few times throughout this process. I hated that the only thing standing in my way were people who weren't listening, people who weren't taking the time to look into the details. It's the same way I used to cry when I had to leave the pharmacy without the medication I needed to live because I couldn't figure out how to get my insurance to be run through correctly. They weren't sad tears. They were pissed. They came from overwhelm and frustration. But as I've practiced being my own advocate, over and over again, I've gotten more used to fighting through the frustrations, fighting through the seemingly endless answers of 'no' until I get to a 'yes.'

It doesn't matter where we learn that resilience - it can be taken from and applied to so many situations. Maybe you've had a well-meaning family member or friend tell you that if you just tried this new raw-food, cinnamon tablet, boiled okra, whatever-the-hell-else concoction that they heard about from their little sister's boss's cousin, you would feel better and be able to participate in more social gatherings (you know, since it's not nice that you've been missing so many of them). Infuriating, huh?

By sticking up for yourself in those situations, by either being very clear about why they have it wrong or by choosing to walk away and not let it bother you, you are practicing being your own advocate. You are choosing to do what you need to do for yourself, for your own mental and physical health, rather than letting someone else tell you what you should or shouldn't be doing.

Knowing that, what other situations do you think you could be applying this bad-ass-ness to?

It's a common joke in our community that anyone diagnosed with a chronic disease should also receive an honorary medical and research doctorate, because the level of knowledge it requires is incomparable. In Malcolm Gladwell's book *Outliers*, he posits that it takes 10,000 hours of practice to become an expert in any subject. One year has 8,760 hours. Hm. And how many years have you been living with your chronic disease? If you don't consider yourself an expert in anything, maybe it's time to reconsider and use your expertise to your advantage.

Ariana Huffington, a highly-educated media mogul, business woman, writer, and politician who holds a degree in economics, is currently best known for her advocacy and research for what? Something she has NO academic or professional expertise in. Sleep.

In 2007, Ariana regularly got about three to four hours of sleep a night. After a whirl-wind college tour with her daughter, where she would regularly stay awake most of the night to work, then spend her days touring campuses, she returned to her home in New York and collapsed on the floor. She ended up breaking her cheekbone, waking up in a pool of her own blood, and requiring stitches. She thought there must be some drastic underlying condition but at the end of months of diagnostics, it was determined. She was suffering from burnout and sleep deprivation.

First, she became an expert. She chose to dive into the study of what supported her health and well-being and, by doing so, became a rallying cry for self-care from an unlikely source. She was a woman who worked 24/7 building a business empire and all of a sudden her message was simple, but went against what so many of the 'sleep when you die' business moguls practiced – instead, rest. Her need to support her own health created her rise to expert-status in a field in which she has no technical training or formal study. She needed to be an expert for herself, so she became an expert. Then after becoming an expert, she became an advocate; not only for herself, but for people across the world who were running themselves into the ground with work. In the offices of The Huffington Post, there are hammocks in the newsroom and bookable nap rooms, as well as breathing and meditation classes. No longer is her experience with sleep deprivation only about her. Like we all can do, she took something that she dealt with, learned about it, shared what she learned, stood up for herself, became an advocate for herself, and became an advocate for others.

Obviously Ariana was already a known figure – by the time she released *Thrive* in 2015 and *The Sleep Revolution* in 2016, she had already been a best-selling author for four decades. She attended Cambridge University, has run for political office, and her website The Huffington Post sold to AOL in 2011 for more than $300 million. She had a few applicable skills before her health taught her a few more. But something she certainly was not an expert in was balance, so the fact that her entire public platform is based upon it now is interesting. She dove into a new subject, was willing to work to learn everything she could about it, unequivocally knows her stuff about everything to do with rest, balance, and well-being in the workplace, refuses to accept anything other than sleep being a vital part of our well-being, and she is willing to fight to spread that message.

It's the same for all of us, really.

Kris Carr, who released Crazy Sexy Cancer Tips in 2007 after her own cancer diagnosis, has taken a similar path of diagnosis to student to expert to advocate. Kris was an actress and photographer (and self-proclaimed party girl) living in New York City when a yoga class didn't provide her usual relief from what she thought was a hangover. After visiting the doctor, she found out that her liver was covered in tumors – she had cancer.

She began writing and filming about her journey while doing everything within her power to do cancer her way. She didn't want to be a science experiment and she didn't feel as though Western medicine's approach of chemotherapy and radiation was right for her, so she became her own advocate. She started doing research on other ways to help herself, other ways to thrive despite and with her cancer.

I know you know what that feels like. There is an odd mixture of dread and meek empowerment that enters your body when you know you're about to tell a trained medical professional that you're not going to take their advice. That you're going to approach this your own way.

If the reactions have been anything like what I've received, you could've gotten anything from a blank stare and silence for a truly uncomfortable amount of time to a sheer dismissal. I'd been given and prescribed the same medication countless times over the course of YEARS before having a doctor finally accept that I just was not going to take it (and thank everything, because that medication was later proved to be quite toxic). It is hard enough telling anyone you're going to take a holistic approach to cancer now – in the early 2000s, I can only imagine that Kris was forced to deal with a fair amount of ridicule. But she stood her ground, continued to research what she felt was right for her, found a care team who respected her decisions, and now has relationships with doctors who work with her to find non-invasive methods to care for her whole mind and body, not just the parts with cancer.

She got creative (she even wore cowboy boots into her first MRI), was willing to work, delving through mountains of information to find answers that worked for her, was steadfast in what she knew, has continued to be stubborn in the kindest, rainbow-unicorn way (I promise that will make sense if you start poking around her YouTube videos - she is delightful), refuses to do this whole cancer thing in any way but her own, and from it all, has created an empire of wellness, helping millions of people not only with cancer, but who were just looking for ways to feel a bit better. She's also become buddies with Oprah and continues to kick cancer's giant backside.

The resilience of learning to be your own advocate is a very real thing. I know that living with chronic disease takes up a lot of your energy, but what do you want to be doing with the rest of it? How can you take this self-advocacy super power and apply it to what you love? You are downright overqualified, honestly. You already know how to do the work - you've always had to with your own health. Take it, reapply it. You already know how.

VISION

L ike many people, I did not have the calmest home life growing up. My father left when I was about three and my mom
got remarried shortly afterward. That marriage wasn't always the most stable, and by the time I was in high school
it was close to over.

When my mom and ex-step-dad were still trying to salvage
their marriage, they started seeing a counselor named Duke.
When I was 17, Duke asked if I would come in for counseling
as well. We were back home in Hawaii after a several year stint
in Washington state, my older brother was living outside of
Seattle on his own, and my little brother was only five and not
fully aware of what was going on with our family. As the kid
who was being most affected by the impending divorce, Duke
wanted to check in with me and see what was happening from
my perspective.

I wasn't very open to this – the few times I had been sent
to a counselor before had been health related, when doctors

or my mom were worried that I wasn't paying close enough attention to keeping my T1D in check. So the idea of going to another counselor to talk things through seemed pointless to me, particularly when it was about something that was outside the realm of what I could control.

After listening to what all was going on and how things were at home from my perspective, Duke said something that has stuck with me since: "don't be distracted by your reality." He encouraged me to do what I needed to do to keep myself sane and safe, continue to write and vent in my giant red journal with my red pen as catharsis, spend time doing anything that brought me joy, and pursue my wish to leave home for college, where I could delve into my own world rather than barring myself against what had become my world at home.

As I've continued to live with chronic disease, I've realized that the concept of not being distracted by reality is something that people who live with constant health challenges are incredibly adept at doing. It's not always what's expected, and I think it may not even be how we, ourselves, always frame it.

I think in most cases, a "better" approach might be to choose to see the good side of something, or figure out how to embrace something negative to turn it into a positive. I actually took a class once, during a time I was struggling in a particularly massive way with my diabetes, about approaching disease with mindfulness. We were taught to sit quietly with each step necessary to take care of ourselves. I don't know about you, but when I'm injecting myself with medicine or pricking myself with a needle for a blood test, sitting with it mindfully is just about the last thing I will choose to do.

Distraction with something better is far more helpful for me, and I think it is for many of us. And I don't at all think it's a bad thing to choose to be distracted by the good in life rather than be distracted by the not so good. If I can chat with a friend as I'm doing a blood test or turn on my favorite show while I'm updating all of my medical supplies, that's far more preferable.

When all is said and done, our reality is what we make it, and we know that. We don't have a choice about whether or not we live with disease, but we choose what to pay attention to, what we allow to shape us, and what we carry forward into the rest of our lives.

Because at the end of the day, our reality of being sick isn't going to become a sparkly positive. It's just not a great thing. And that's okay. Nothing in life is made up of all great things, and the true superpower comes in not being distracted by the lackluster stuff that comes with being human.

If you've ever seen me from behind (stick with me here) you'll know that I have a Deathly Hallows tattoo on the base of my neck (see, we made it to a not so weird place after all!). If you have no idea what the Deathly Hallows are, put this book down and go read or watch the 7th installment of Harry Potter. I'll wait.

The first Harry Potter book was released in the US in June of 1997, five months before I was diagnosed with T1D. A new book was released every few years until 2007, when the final book was released during the summer between my sophomore and junior years in college. Every single one of us staying on campus that summer had ordered *Harry Potter and the Deathly Hallows* on Amazon to arrive at our dorms on its release date and none of us spoke for 24 hours after the mail came that day. We were twenty years old and voraciously reading the final volume with as much gusto as each of us had read the rest.

Those books were my companions through my diagnosis, through challenging times with my family, through leaving home to go 6,000 miles away to a place I had never been to go to school, through heartbreaks and health scares and the general challenge of growing up. And they would not exist had J.K. Rowling chosen to be distracted by her own reality.

In the early 1990s, J.K., also known as Jo, had just moved to Scotland after going through a divorce. She and her young child were near destitute, she was on unemployment, and she was battling a major clinical depression. After having come up with the idea for Harry Potter on a train ride, she decided that nothing could be lost by trying. That if every major publishing house rejected her book, she would be no worse off than she already was. And so she wrote. The world she created went on to be the best selling book series of all time (with more than 447 million copies sold), was made into the best selling movie series of all time (with almost $8 billion (yes, with a 'b') in box office revenue), and was turned into an existing, physical world by Universal Studios. And butterbeer was created in reality, and all was good in the world.

No one would have blamed Jo for putting off writing to take care of herself. She was worried about her own well-being, as well as the well-being of her child. There were things she could have chosen to take care of first – to wait until things were more stable, to wait until she was feeling stronger, to wait until her daughter was older. She could have allowed herself to slowly heal, but instead she hunkered down and dove into her work, her own little world that she had created. Her reality was not her limitation. She lived in her imagined world and by doing so, is one of the most successful writers of all time. She created an alternate reality that comforts people, reminds us of the power of friendship, and inspires courage in the face of seemingly insurmountable odds.

That's what I think is incredibly cool about all of us living with this not so great health stuff – we choose to go tackle the big things anyway. So many people never chase what they really want to go after. They allow the distractions of their current situations to hold them back from amazing things.

But you've learned that when you're feeling sick, one of the best things you can do for yourself is to not be distracted by it, to go do something that you wanted to do anyway, even if it means tweaking it a bit to accommodate for whatever is going on in your life right now and however you're feeling. Do you know how many people literally never learn to do that?

Your disease will always be present in your life, but more often than not, you're choosing not to be distracted by it or overwhelmed by it, or allowing it to hold you back. (For the record, yes we ALL have times when these feelings hit us upside the head, but we don't allow them to hunker down and stay).

How do I know that you're choosing all of that? You're reading this book. There are so many people who allow themselves to wallow, to completely sink into their sickness, and I honestly cannot judge them for it. I have so much compassion for people who are completely lost in being sick. It is such a hard thing to choose to come out of.

But you're here. Something in you already recognized that you have great things to bring to the world and you just need to figure out how to not let your health get in the way. See? Superpowers.

When my mom was going through what ended up being a several-year path toward divorce, she had mantra cards that she kept with her. One of them said, "It has been so long since something bad has happened that I've forgotten what it feels like to be afraid."

It is a scary thing to feel like the ground is going to fall out from under you at any moment. To know, in the back of your mind, that this illness you carry with you can interrupt at any time. That you can experience a flare-up, that a treatment won't work as planned, that you forgot a medication at an inopportune time and ended up having to make a plane turn around over the ocean to rush back to the closest hospital before you slipped into a coma from a stupid packing mistake (guilty).

It is a challenge of the utmost courage to forge ahead anyway, to accept your illness while not allowing it to limit you, to choose to set those fears aside, and do the thing. But you are better for it. You are stronger for it. Your dream can only happen in direct proportion to your courage, and you are so incredibly capable of it.

The first few days I spent as an inpatient at Seattle Children's Hospital after my diagnosis, I had a roommate named Sarah. Sarah had a degenerative muscle disease, was limited to her bed, and couldn't eat food on her own. She got her calories and nutrients from little bottles of Ensure, which were poured into her stomach tube. She was bubbly and hilarious. She always had jokes to tell, and always had a smile on her face. I don't think she was much older than eleven or twelve.

Once I was more medically stable and therefore a little more mobile, I was allowed to wander down to the hospital's cafeteria with my mom, IV in tow, robe tightly wrapped around me. On our first venture out, we ran into Sarah's mom in the dining room. She was exhausted. They had flown down from Alaska, where they lived, for Sarah to come to the children's hospital for treatment. Sarah wasn't doing well. Her mom wasn't entirely sure how this visit was going to end up.

My mom started asking Sarah's mom about her favorite stories from Sarah's younger years. A few years prior, when Sarah was still healthy enough to attend regular school days, she decided to bring in her roller blades for show and tell. Sarah was using a walker by that point, but still loved to roller blade down the sidewalk by slowly pushing her walker in front of herself as she rolled along.

On this particular day in school, she somehow convinced her teachers that wearing her roller blades made it easier for her to get to classes, rather than having to slowly shuffle through the hallway. That transformed into Sarah rallying a small group of kids to have a race, which quickly became Sarah going as fast as she could down the hallway, rollerblades on, helmet strapped, walker skidding along the floor. Sarah ended up falling and knocking out her two front teeth on her walker. She got up laughing. She had had a blast.

Sarah was always trying to find ways to have more fun, to inspire more laughter, to do new things. Her body was failing her, but she wasn't letting it distract her from experiencing joy and having fun. It was a courageous choice - to choose happiness in the face of her very real, very scary situation.

If you have spent any time on the internet in the past few years, you've probably seen some videos with Kid President (if you haven't, go look up "A Pep Talk from Kid President to You"). He's the amazingly charming and energetic kid, forever in a suit, who talks to us about "treating everybody like it's their birthday" and "giving the world a reason to dance." He also makes incredibly astute observations like, "give people high fives for getting out of bed. Being a person is hard sometimes."

It would be easy to write off Kid President, whose actual name is Robby Novak, as a carefully produced product of the YouTube culture, but what's amazing is that the entire Kid President THING was a project done in Tennessee with Robby and his older brother-in-law Brad Montague because they liked being creative and making things with each other. Brad believes that kids have important things to say and share, Robby always has messages to share with us all, and thus Kid President was born.

And here's the amazing thing - Robby has the genetic disorder osteogenesis imperfecta, which means his bones are extremely susceptible to damage. By the time he was ten, Robby had already experienced more than 70 bone fractures. And he's giving US pep talks.

That's the key, I think. Because we live with these realities that are sometimes painful, sometimes nauseating, sometimes exhausting, almost always emotionally draining, and sometimes all of those things at the same time, plus whatever else we're faced with, we have to fight through it to get to this place of building, creativity, and production. I would venture to say that

that only inspires further greatness on the other side. We know what we're fighting through. It's not like we're living in a fairy-tale world where we think everything is fine and we don't know what we're facing. But it makes us know why it's worth it – why it's worth gathering ourselves up to take the first steps toward a big goal. Why it's worth fighting through a particularly hard day to finish a special project. It turns into a drive like no one else has.

IMPERFECTION

Despite all of our drive and general gung-ho nature, we know we cannot attain perfection. We're reminded of this more often than others. While other people are berating themselves for not being perfect, not having the perfect body, not having the perfect social life, not having the perfect personality, we forgive ourselves for much more basic things – not having the energy to be the cool party-girl we feel like people want us to be, our medical results not coming back at the levels we wanted them to be, only being able to do half of the workout we had planned. Because we must forgive ourselves. It is the only way we can survive in a life where our health is not always cooperating.

What an amazing weight off our shoulders that is. Perfectionism holds you back, it does not propel you forward. Fighting your imperfections will only wear you out and break you down. We know this fact more than others ever have to learn, but that in itself is such an amazing thing. Embracing our imperfections leads to a level of conscious self-love that is imperative for our own well-being.

It's about not beating yourself up when you make a mistake, but loving yourself through the mistakes, of which there will be many. None of us are immune to mistakes. On the other side of this self-love is grace, is confidence - the tools it takes to be great, to stand strong, and to have the courage to chase everything you want, because you know you can, and you're perfectly okay with the imperfections you'll meet along the way.

And of course with that level of self-love comes higher levels of self-confidence, which has been particularly tied to women being able to attain more leadership roles, start their own successful companies, and create powerful platforms to improve others' lives. Blazing your own trail requires you to be okay with your imperfections, to know that they're going to come along for the ride, and to know that they can actually teach you and inform your approach to challenges. Knowing and loving your imperfections lets you accommodate for them.

Luckily this idea of trying to not be quite so obsessed with perfection has become a bit more mainstream over the past few years. In the early 2010s, articles started sprouting up saying it just wasn't possible to be perfect at absolutely everything and women really needed to stop trying, lest we run ourselves into the ground. They recognized that women were expected to work a 60-hour work week at a promising start up while simultaneously leaving work early enough to pick up her kids from the best prep school in the area, while also looking like a model and having enough time to work out and eat like one, while also maintaining the perfect home life, and so on. It's a really great thing we knew this already, because the thought-pieces on this topic are numerous enough that it's no secret it's something huge amounts of women were struggling with. When we don't believe that we, just as we are, are enough, we start to crumble.

Drew Barrymore, the actress you know from movies like "E.T.", the modern "Charlie's Angels" movies, and "The Wedding Singer", among others, has been incredibly vocal about this, and how the very real pressure to be perfect can be damaging. After a very public battle with alcoholism, drug use, and mental health all before she was a teenager, she stayed in the movie business and, some years, was simultaneously producing, directing, and acting in several movies. She loved film, but coming from an actor family put on its own set of pressures about success and perfectionism in an already tough industry. While she appreciated being able to pour herself into what she loved, in a 2016 interview with Harper's Bazaar she said, "I think it's a huge mistake to think you have to burn bright for your whole life. You cannot sustain it. It's exhausting, and it's not very realistic."

Now, having stepped back a bit from her life as an actress, she splits her days between being a full-time mom and working on her own passion projects. She said it's rare that she ever does both at the same time – when she's in mom-mode, she just focuses on being a mom. When the kids are otherwise occupied, she focuses on her creative projects. Rather than trying to be all things at all times, she just focuses on being present, not perfect. She's been able to publish two books over the last few years, has her own makeup line and wine company, and is able to delve into her love of photography. She doesn't do any of it because she's perfect at it; she does it all because it makes her happy. It is her way of loving herself.

When you're dealing with struggles with your health, you require even more self love. There are times when we want to be able to shove our sickness aside so we can run toward our goals, but accepting that our bodies are working as hard as they can and loving on ourselves for all that we do is so crucial. It allows us to approach our goals creatively, figuring out how to still make them happen, just like Drew has, because we love what we're doing, not because we feel like we have to be the absolute best in everything that we try.

One of my favorite TED Talks of all time is with a woman named Maysoon Zayid. Maysoon, a Palestinian-American stand-up comedian from New Jersey, co-founded the New York Arab-American Comedy Festival. When she's not doing stand up, she spends a few months of her year in Palestine, where she teaches disabled and orphaned children art to help deal with trauma.

Throughout everything she does, the stand-up comedy, the art workshops abroad, and her everyday life, Maysoon must sit often, and she never stops shaking. Her body is always moving in violent little jerks. It's a result of her cerebral palsy (CP), an outcome not of a disease or birth defect, but of her near suffocation at birth brought upon by a delivery that was performed by a drunk doctor.

There are certain things in life that I think people absolutely deserve to be really angry about. Living with CP because of someone else's utter carelessness is one of them. But Maysoon instead approaches everything she does with wit, humor, and an immense amount of self-love.

She's not shy about her CP – she can't be, as her shakes are so visible – but she could have chosen to be angry. She could have chosen to hate this side of herself. I don't doubt that there are times when she's frustrated with it. But instead she's turned it into not only a platform to connect with others, but as a way to pay it forward to other children who are going through trauma, and as a way to advocate for equal and accurate representation of minorities in media.

Not only that, but her own passion and love for herself, rather than being ashamed or angry about her condition, has led to her ability to start a world renowned comedy festival that has been running for more than a decade. The New York Arab-American Comedy Festival is vital; not only is it providing a needed platform for talented comedians, writers, directors, actors, and filmmakers, but it is also creating access. Its reach, along with its growing coverage by the media, is exposing our culture and the entertainment industry to a more diverse representation of Arab-Americans in media. This could not have happened without Maysoon first embracing herself, the many sides of herself, so that she could help bring this to us.

What I learn most from Maysoon is this – what could hold you back never has to. It's not the rule that someone living with CP cannot do stand-up comedy, cannot travel to help others, cannot be in Adam Sandler movies (for real, she has!), and cannot do amazing things. If anything, the skills learned from the challenges Maysoon lives with instead informed her decisions to work harder and be a louder advocate for people like her.

Embracing these imperfections – the things you live with that challenge you, whatever they are – is what teaches you a special level of self-love that is the link to being a powerful leader and voice in your community. You know that your imperfections don't take away from your abilities. Instead, embracing and even publicly acknowledging them helps people embrace you. It makes you more accessible, more real, more trustworthy. In turn, your example helps other people learn to embrace themselves. It's this beautiful little kumbaya circle, and you get to start it.

Who better to look to as the ultimate example of this than the mother of all things herself, Oprah. I was a teenager when Oprah was going through her seemingly never-ending and very public battle with her weight. She was constantly yo-yo dieting and her journey with her body was the focus of extreme public scrutiny. It seemed like every time I went to the grocery store with my mom, unflattering pictures of Oprah were plastered across tabloids, alongside did-she-didn't-she stories of extreme weight loss methods and callous remarks about whether or not Oprah deserved to be an example of women empowerment when she couldn't manage her own body.

Oprah has never been shy about what was going on at that point - she has since said that her weight gain was a direct result of emotional turmoil from poor relationships. She never felt like she was quite good enough in her intimate relationships and it led to a major personal struggle of worthiness, translating into a lack of alignment within herself that threw her body into imbalance. She was hard on herself, and she suffered for it. She needed others' approval, and it deprived her of the self-love she needed to be her happiest, healthiest self.

She was absolutely already successful at that point. The Oprah Winfrey Show had been on the air since 1986 and to this day remains the highest-rated talk show in American television history. But something very interesting started happening in the first decade of the 2000s. O, The Oprah Magazine was first published in April 2000. In it, she writes a monthly column, What I Know For Sure (which she later turned into a book of compiled columns, published in 2014). She bares her heart in these columns. She tells us of her struggles, her mistakes, her side steps. All of the times she thought she was going to fail. All of the times she did fail. She tells us of her breakdowns and freak-outs. She then goes on to explain what each of these episodes taught her, and how each learning experience allowed her to step into a new and better place. She is imperfect, and it gives us hope.

Oprah's level of self-love had shifted, and being who she was, we all got to watch it happen. As she learned to further embrace herself, struggles, flaws, and all, her reach and influence expanded almost beyond the imaginable. Whereas in the late 1990s, she was highly influential but still talked about relentlessly for not being thin enough, engaging enough, or worthy of her success, her constant and dogged chase of recognizing and embracing her own truths led to something almost super-human. After a slow start, the OWN network, launched in 2011, was Oprah's largest and most recent major venture. It is now broadcast in more than 70% of American households.

From a young woman who struggled with self-image and with loving herself through abusive relationships, she is now considered to be the most influential woman in the world. "The Oprah Effect," jokingly named, is the not at all made-up effect of what happens when Oprah mentions your product, platform, or message. Her influence is so large that she can launch people to extreme success with a single mention. As of this book's publication, she is worth almost four billion dollars and is both one of the richest self-made women in America, as well as one of the most philanthropic. All from a woman who has publicly battled, at length, with her own imperfections, then learned to love and accept them, turning that self-love into a launch pad of her entire brand. It was when Oprah learned to love herself more that she found higher levels of success and acceptance.

Sometimes we have to learn this self-love the hard way. I know that I get sick often, and that sometimes my body just shuts down. I could get angry that I can't always do work like others, that I can't pull all-nighters or live off of donuts and coffee. Instead, those times when my body needs me to step aside for a moment are the perfect times for me to show myself a little extra love. It's in that down-time, that time when I'm not chasing perfection, that I'm actually able to realign and make sure I'm on the right path. I end up figuring out how to maximize my time creatively. I get highly organized. I figure out what tools I need to fill in the gaps where I just can't be. And none of that is from any particular place of great skill – it's from necessity.

If you're nodding along here, which I'm willing to bet you are, you know how much our lives require this. Even with decreased time, we tend not to do less. Our knowledge of our imperfection – knowing that our system is just going to fade out sometimes – has led to the skill of extreme efficiency. There is a certain confidence in our ability to get something done once we learn that our imperfections don't have to be a set-back. And there is a certain superpower in loving ourselves enough to know that perfectionism is never necessary; we are fine just the way we are.

PURPOSE

Another form of perfectionism is the feeling of having to say "yes" to everything and anything that anyone expects or asks of you. But anyone who lives with any kind of health issues has to get really good at "no." Without that magic little word in our arsenal, we run the risk of taking on way too much outside of what our energy stores allow. To be clear, this doesn't necessarily have to mean that we have less energy than your everyday person, but it does mean that we get more painful reminders that we've overexerted ourselves when we stretch a bit too far.

Being able to say no to the onslaught of more opportunities, more things to do, more obligations, etc. is a way of honoring yourself, of listening to your body and your intuition. It may feel like you're missing out on things sometimes - particularly in our age of everything being shown on social media, there's a very in-your-face constant reminder of things that you turned down. And of course for any overachiever there's a certain amount of, "Oh no, what have I done?!" that comes after turning down an opportunity. It doesn't matter if you don't have time. It doesn't matter if it doesn't align with your goals or your focus. A turned down opportunity feels like a particular kind of failure, because we're the kind of people who can typically take on a lot and do it well.

But with both our health and our goals, learning how to say no to the things that are not 100% right for us is a true skill. It's almost like we're front loading the lesson. Inevitably, those who say yes to far too many things, spreading themselves incredibly thin, are the same people who end up crashing later in life, keeling over from heart attacks in the prime of their business or, like in Ariana Huffington's case, passing out in the middle of the day from exhaustion.

A quick online search will tell you a myriad of stories of business people who pushed themselves too hard, never taking a break, never putting up boundaries, ultimately leading to major health issues or even death. One of the sad stories of the last few years was a young German intern named Moritz Erhardt, who was doing a several week internship in London for Bank of America Merrill Lynch's international investment bank division. Over the course of two weeks, he had pulled eight all-nighters; the company was notorious for expecting interns and people who were otherwise proving themselves to stay late. After three all-nighters in a row, Moritz passed out and died in his shower. Another intern, after Moritz's death, stated in a Daily Mail article that "About 100 hours a week was the minimum and the average was probably 110. I worked six-and-a-half days a week."

What's sad to me is that these interns didn't feel like they could say no. They felt that in order to achieve, they had to put up with outlandish requests to stay at work past the point of any kind of healthy expectation.

For better or worse, I have become particularly good at no. Honestly, it's not always appreciated, particularly in work situations when a boss has felt like she should be getting 80 hours of work a week out of a young person. I have always been very clear that I don't work into the evenings and weekends unless it's for pre-planned events, and other people's lack of planning never constitutes my emergency. Because let's face it, nothing I do is important enough that it's saving lives minute-to-minute and therefore nothing I do is important enough to sacrifice my own health by pushing too hard. Saying no and setting my own boundaries around what I do and when I do it has never held me back from achieving and doing exactly what I wanted professionally, and it's certainly never held me back in any of my own projects. The key, which I'm sure you've experienced, is making sure the no is coming from a place of self-care, rather than a place of fear.

The reality is, no matter what held you back from saying yes from a place of self-care to an opportunity – a particularly bad health flare, just not having enough time, knowing you needed to prioritize something else – sometimes a part of you feels like the only actual reason you couldn't take advantage of the opportunity was because you weren't good enough to manage it. You feel like you've thrown something away that you'll never find again. You become worried that the thing you passed up could have been your big break. You missed it. It's gone. You may as well get used to a subpar life, because that's what it's going to be from now on.

But of course, once you come back from that little fear-based moment, you know that's not how this all works. You know that what's for you will always find you again. If it's not the right timing for you, then it's not the right thing for you. You already know that just because you've had to say no to an opportunity does not mean another never came your way. As icky as it feels sometimes in the moment, you've learned that turning some things down doesn't make you any less capable than anyone else. It actually means you know how to prioritize, and that in itself is a skill.

We already know how to say no, and that, my dear, is a superpower. It's often said that saying yes to something means saying no to something else. So often, and for so many peo-ple, constantly saying yes to every new shiny opportunity that passes their way actually means saying no to sleep, to a project that would have been much more in alignment with what they actually enjoy doing, to seeing their family, to getting to spend a quiet Saturday evening with friends and a few bottles of wine, laughing for hours at a time.

Those people who don't know how to say no, they're actually inadvertently saying no to a lot of things that really matter. They just don't know it yet.

And that's where our superpower comes into play. It feels sucky to have to pass on opportunities sometimes, but in reality, there is not a single human on this planet who can take on every single thing that comes her way. We are not machines. We're humans, and humans need care. We need breaks. We need priorities. The people who don't realize that soon enough are, ironically in this case, the ones who end up running themselves straight into sickness, brought upon by never figuring out how to slow down and figure out what needs to be number one in their lives.

It's weird, but by having this health challenge first, we are forced to learn this skill. The realization that you get to pick and choose what's best for you, that you're not supposed to take on every single thing that comes your way, is going to save you a lot of exhaustion and burnout later.

Sheryl Sandberg, COO of Facebook and former VP at Google, is famous for something very particular that she does – she leaves work every day at 5:30pm. It wasn't until her book Lean In and the growth of its accompanying foundation that she even spoke about this publicly, since the expectation at so many high-achieving companies is to stay until later hours of the evening, at least.

Particularly in Silicon Valley, known for entrepreneurs who sleep under their desks, working for days on end without showering to get a huge project out the door, saying no to that kind of rat race can sometimes be unheard of. For a massive business leader like Sheryl, it's not that she doesn't have plenty she could be doing into the wee hours of the night; it's that she's prioritizing also having time with her family, and having time for herself.

Clearly it's not gotten in the way of her massive success. You cannot count on one hand how many times she's been named to Fortune Magazine's 50 Most Powerful Women in Business list. Her entire foundation is based upon the idea that women should press harder for their success and not be afraid to be strong voices in the workplace. But she's also never said that this requires saying yes to every single opportunity in order to become known as the person who can do it all. Very strongly, she instead says that success is about the expectations we set for ourselves and how we demand to be seen and treated by others. No is clearly not a weakness when it comes to business, and it's certainly not a weakness in other incredibly important aspects of our life as well.

We all got to learn this lesson in Elizabeth Gilbert's *Eat, Pray, Love*. Liz walked away from something - a marriage in her case – that wasn't necessarily bad, it just wasn't right for her.

Interestingly enough, that's also what she got the most backlash for from the story she shared with us. People were so angry that she said "no" to something good. But walking away from something that one could argue is good enough takes an incredible amount of courage.

It is so easy to convince ourselves that the thing in front of us is good (and that we might never find something that good again), so we would be incredibly stupid not cling to it with a resounding "yes." What we don't always have the courage to realize is that the good thing isn't always the right thing.

When Liz got brave enough to walk away, it's not that she wasn't scared of what was coming next. It's not that she wasn't going to have breakdowns. She went through periods of thinking she must be utterly insane. It's the absolute same steps we all go through when we say no to an opportunity – denial, shame, fear, doubt. She walked away from stability, a home, and a husband to travel the world and focus on finding what was truly right for her. She hadn't had a bad life, but she hadn't had the right life for her.

She traveled through Italy, India, and Bali. She ultimately found her people, and certainly found an incredible level of success. Liz had been a writer for her entire life. She had already had articles, short story collections, a novel, and a biography published. But it wasn't until the courage of telling her story in *Eat, Pray, Love* that Liz found her current level of success (complete with her book being made into a movie starring Julia Roberts). She had the courage to say no to her current life (despite the criticism she faced, externally and internally), the courage to pursue what was right for her, and the courage to really trust her gut to only accept what was truly in alignment with the life she wanted.

She didn't do a whirlwind trip of every country. She didn't send herself into a high-achieving frenzy. She was deliberate. She said no to hundreds of other places that would have been perfectly wonderful places to go to. She said no to that distraction. She chose what she needed for herself in that moment.

It's not just massive life decisions that this applies to – as I write this book, my mom is in the process of launching her brick and mortar wellness center in coastal South Carolina, Second Wind Therapy & Wellness. The center is particularly focused on helping people with movement and neurological disorders, typically older people dealing with things like Parkinsons, people who are trying to recover from debilitating accidents, or veterans dealing with trauma.

My mom and I also own an online wellness business together, where we help people use nutrition as a path toward health, whether their goals are weight loss, sports performance, or just general well-being. To be completely honest, my mom has been carrying the weight of that business for a while. I've been choosing to focus on other things that are speaking to me a bit more right now (hi, book), but soon I know I'll step in more so that she can focus on her wellness center. It's all an ebb and flow.

My mom and I have carefully cultivated our communication over the years, so I know that this situation is not necessarily one that everyone gets to enjoy, but halfway through my writing this chapter, my mom reached out to me to ask if I could step in a bit more with our online social forum for our customers, a place where we share information on nutrition, answer questions, and help people through their health conundrums. In the past, I've really loved helping moderate this platform. I love to jump in and help people who are going through the kinds of puzzles I've been through with my own health, that I was only able to solve with nutritional help. But I told her, very honestly, that I was at capacity with my other projects and I just was not going to have time right now. To be honest, I absolutely felt like a bit of a jerk for saying no. We all have that gut reaction. Her response? "I thought that might be the case and I am super grateful you are honest about your boundaries/limits!"

It's something that can only be learned by doing it - people generally appreciate your saying "you know what, it just doesn't fit into my priorities right now." Think about it - how many times have you been frustrated working with a colleague or fellow student on a group project because they showed up all excited at the start of a project but then went ghost? How much more helpful is it to work with someone who, from the start, has a clear idea of what she's going to be able to contribute, what her time constraints are, and what a reasonable expectation can be for the outcome. How much stress does that save us all?

By having a good pulse on what you're willing to spend time on (and therefore what you're not), you actually help everyone. If someone asks us to spend the weekend marathoning our way through a project and we respond with, "you know what, I actually tend to crash on weekends, but I'd be more than happy to help you put this together over the course of a few Tuesday afternoons," we are being incredibly helpful to others. Our skill of saying no, even if it makes us cringe a little bit sometimes (if it doesn't make you cringe, hip hip hooray! I'm proud of you), not only helps us but helps others plan for success as well.

I recently read a profile of a woman named Saiyyidah Zaidi, who walked away from a program director job in the United Kingdom that paid $170,000 a year. In her position, she had managed a £500 million budget and oversaw fifty staffers. She had spent her whole life working toward an executive director role and walked away when she was about to reach it, realizing she didn't want it anymore.

In her rise to the top, she was putting in long hours away from her family, working within an organization whose decisions she did not always agree with. Her household went from a six-figure salary to her husband's $25,000 per year overnight. She had the courage to say no to something that looked really great, but she knew wasn't right for her.

She knew she excelled at coaching people; in her old position, she loved serving as a mentor to her employees. So instead of saying yes to the traditional opportunities that had been coming her way – a woman who knew how to manage both such a large budget and that many people had organizations trying to knock down her door to get her – she decided to only say yes to anything that aligned with this new vision of what she actually enjoyed and where she felt she could truly give back. She now coaches fellow Muslim women on how to start their own business and is able to provide microfinance loans to women in the developing world. By saying no to something in which she was truly excelling at, she not only found her passion, but is able to bring valuable services to a worthy group of women who needed her help.

One of my favorite people on the planet is a young woman named Peta Kelly. She is an Australian spitfire whose every sentence contains a cuss word (it's the Aussie way, after all) and leads with her heart in literally every single thing she does.

She's a self-made millionaire in her late 20s, but just a few years ago she was earning $500 a week while pursuing her PhD in exercise sciences. She was fascinated by the human body and figured becoming a professor would help her reach her goal of making enough money to support both herself and her mum, a single mother of four who had provided Peta and her brother and sisters everything she could while also being a teacher herself.

One day Peta wandered into her PhD advisor's office in tears. She knew in her gut that she wasn't going down the right path for her. She didn't know what the right path was yet, but she had the courage to say no to a continued pursuit of her PhD to figure out what it was.

This is something that I think is really key in our journeys with ourselves – part of being able to say no at the right moments is being incredibly in touch with ourselves. I think part of the magic of being someone who lives with chronic disease is that I know my body better than anything else I know in the world. We all live with our bodies for our entire lives, and yet so many people don't know how to listen to them.

Intuition and alignment give us literal gut feelings. The chemicals that balance our brain are primarily made in the gut, so when we know something isn't quite right, that's why we don't just feel it in our minds. It is spread throughout our body. When it's time to say no, being so in touch with our own bodies, because we've been through hell with each other, is an exceedingly helpful thing. We've learned to listen in the moments where others might ignore.

After walking away from her PhD, Peta spent the next few years getting involved with a health and wellness company, coaching people toward better health, and ultimately becoming one of the top earners in her space. Her journey has brought her into a space of working with hundreds of other generation y leaders, young people who are doing seriously impressive things in the world, paving the way for higher thinking, more success, and more giving back to their communities.

Peta runs several projects, events, and coaching groups, all aimed at helping young people figure out what lights them up and how to share that with others. She helps people bring their unique gifts to the world by helping them figure out how to tune in to what they can offer the world that aligns with what the world needs. Her intuition and connection with herself, the superpowers that led her to originally say no to a perfectly great and noble path, are precisely what got her to where she is now. She would not now be able to mobilize her tribe of conscious young leaders without her original pushback against the opportunity to earn a PhD.

And yes, Peta was called crazy by her friends. One of the toughest stories I've listened to her tell is one where she was absolutely torn to shreds by her former friends on Facebook. One person she knew wrote a public post about how Peta was basically full of it. How, in walking away from the things and opportunities people thought she should be aligned with to pursue something else, people thought she was being fake and a liar. Former friends jumped on to the post, tearing her to shreds. It was a feeding frenzy of jealousy and misunderstanding from a truly miserable group of people.

That's why this particular superpower is courageous. It is not easy to say no. It is not easy to walk away from something good, to doubt yourself and to know that others will doubt you too, so that you can pursue something better.

Sometimes that something better is being able to take care of yourself as you need to or walking away from something good to run toward something better. Sometimes that something better is paving the way for Muslim women who want to start small businesses, or millennials who are using their entrepreneurial skills to bring much needed messages and solutions to the world. Either way, it starts with the courage to first say no. But it's courage you already possess. As Peta says, "you already know the answer, and you get to choose."

The superpower of saying no, which you've learned from a life of having to have it as a tool in your arsenal, is such an important one to lead to success in all aspects of your life. Being able to truly prioritize, to step back and take a look at what the right things are for you to say yes to, is such a profound skill. Many never learn it, but you've already got it tucked away. It's up to you to go use it as a way to figure out exactly what you want to jump at, to say yes to, and exactly what deserves a big fat no.

SUPERPOWER #5
QUIRKINESS

Meryl Streep, the actress with an astonishing 19 Academy Award nominations (she's won three), started her career in the New York City theater. After her first audition for a film role, the lead in the 1976 version of King Kong, the Italian director turned to his son and said, "This is so ugly. Why did you bring me *this*?" The director, of course, didn't know that Meryl spoke Italian.

Meryl, for all of her acting talent, was not known as a classic leading lady, nor has she ever been known for playing your average woman character. She plays the interesting characters, the odd ones, the complex ones, the strong ones. Regularly called "our greatest living actress" by the media, she has said, "what makes you different or weird, that's your strength."

What's your strength? Living with chronic disease already sets us apart from the crowd (although, of course, more and more people are being diagnosed with chronic illnesses every day). That doesn't necessarily feel like a strength, though I'm just waiting for the day when these odd health developments actually turn into a legitimate I-can-do-something-useful-with-this mutation.

What is absolutely a strength, however, is the culmination of all the oddball things we've had to learn to best support ourselves through being sick. There aren't a whole lot of people I know who understand their bodies to the level that I do, and I'm betting you could either say the same, or you'll be to that point soon. At a recent doctor's appointment, a physician who was new to my patient file was trying to run through a whole host of possibilities as to why I had been in a particularly large amount of pain and feeling extra fatigued.

"I think it could be that you're not getting enough potassium."

"Nope, that's not it."

"...are you sure? How do you know? We haven't run that blood test yet."

"That's not what this feels like."

"... but how do you know that."

"I just know."

A blood test that day later showed that I actually have more than enough potassium (I have always taken Popeye to heart – I eat a lot of spinach). But the you-are-absolutely-a-weirdo looks I got that day from that doctor are nothing new. I've learned to generally be pretty entertained by them.

I am very used to being seen as the odd one out, not only by medical professionals but by a lot of people in my personal life as well. My friends have embraced it, as friends do. I have one friend who mimics my insulin pump beeps whenever different alarms go off. Strangers get annoyed by the noise; she thinks it's really entertaining that I'm bionic.

But I also get that people tend not to like to accommodate the weird ones all the time. At health food stores, employees get irritated that I'm that picky customer – when offered free samples of whatever super-life-enhancing-coconut-water-smoothie of the day they're selling, I ask for an ingredient list. I know in their minds they're thinking "lady, it's already healthy, what more do you want?" But I can imagine it would not exactly make their day if I had an anaphylactic reaction to one of the random things that sets my immune system off in their store. My being picky actually serves both of us rather well in that situation.

Learning to live with that and being absolutely sure that, at the end of the day, these seemingly outsider decisions you have to make for yourself are what is best for you, teaches you to embrace your weirdness. It gives you a certain level of confidence in your differences that others struggle to achieve. It's yet another superpower.

I've learned to be confident in the fact that there are out-side-of-the-mainstream things that work well for me and my body. Embracing that I am the weird one who believes in energy work, meditation, anti-inflammatory nutrition, listening to the universe, and lots of sleep, among other things, has taught me to stand strong in my convictions, not only with my health, but also in everything I do in life.

Once you learn that, it's a different kind of life. Once you embrace your weird, you get to travel a much less crowded road. While many other people are trying to fit in, you get to fly above. That much less crowded road leaves room for you to explore all the cool things that no one else is doing. It's embracing the weird that leads to new inventions, the next best-selling novel, businesses that changes millions of people's lives, and beautiful masterpieces. None of that could be created by someone who was just trying to be normal, just trying to blend into the crowd.

Having the courage to be the one standing outside of the crowd, particularly when it means taking care of the only body you get to live in and the only mind you get to possess, is a super power typically possessed only by people who went through hell to earn it. There's a good chance you were doing all of the normal stuff before, right? Before you realized you needed to put your health first, you may have partied hard, worked out too little, ate a few things that didn't make you feel the best. And that's fine. I absolutely did it too, even after I was already diagnosed with my primary health issues, because the feeling of "other", of having to stand alone, can be incredibly heavy. But it is the weird ones who really thrive in this world, and by already having to be comfortable being the weird one, you have worked your way into an elite world. We had to earn our way to weird. Embrace it.

We are the nutrition nerds, the ones who are picky about what we consume. We are particular about where we go, who we spend time around, and who we allow to affect our energy. We have limited resources (spoons, to some - hey spoonies!) and we choose to only share those resources with those who have earned them. We choose to do what is best for us, because we don't necessarily have the time or energy to be all things to all people (nor does anyone). If you need a rallying cry to clinch this as a great thing in your mind, I can't think of one much better than the famous Think Different ad for Apple, written by Rob Siltanen and his team at TBWA/Chiat/Day:

"Here's to the crazy ones. The misfits. The rebels. The troublemakers. The round pegs in the square holes. The ones who see things differently. They're not fond of rules. And they have no respect for the status quo. You can quote them, disagree with them, glorify or vilify them. About the only thing you can't do is ignore them. Because they change things. They push the human race forward. And while some may see them as the crazy ones, we see genius. Because the people who are crazy enough to think they can change the world, are the ones who do."

So there you have it – we are the ones who have embraced the weird, embraced the crazy, to do what we need to do for ourselves. In turn, it can provide the motivation for others to be the weird ones too.

And do you know whose crazy company we're in? The special circle of the super weird people like Elon Musk and Lady Gaga, supreme weirdos who have turned their peculiarity and their not giving a damn what others thought into amazing success. Unsurprisingly, once the general public gets over the first few steps, they learn to appreciate the weird. It's like people need to know that you're really serious about the weird - that you've committed to this oddball life. Once they have enough evidence, it's no longer weird, it's visionary.

Lady Gaga, the creative force behind the dress made of deli meat once worn on a red carpet (sometimes creative for the sake of creative is just that – it doesn't have to be a home run knocked out of the park every time), was born Stefani Joanne Angelina Germanotta to hard-working Italian-American parents. She grew up on the Upper West Side of New York City, attending prestigious schools on the Upper East Side. Stefanie was a hard-working, over-achieving student but, as she said, "I used to get made fun of for being either too provocative or too eccentric, so I started to tone it down. I didn't fit in, and I felt like a freak."

After getting into theater and attending performing arts programs and schools, Stefani started rising to prominence in the Lower East Side's avant garde performing arts scene. She was getting better and better known, but still walked the line of freak to so many people. To the avant garde scene, legend has it that she was getting too big, too mainstream. To the mainstream scene, even after she signed a secure record deal, she was too racy, too underground.

It was Gaga, embracing her weird self and getting incredibly sure about her approach being the right approach - that her racy, dance-oriented, pop music was the direction music culture was headed, even if the record executives didn't see that yet - that led her down the path she is on now. As of the start of 2016, she had sold 27 million albums worldwide and become a clear rallying person for so many people who feel like they have to hide, who feel like who they really are is not going to be accepted by their friends, family, and community. Waving her freak flag high, continuing to fully embrace her eccentricities and creativity, has given other people permission to be exactly, unapologetically, who they are.

I can imagine that's something that you're doing for your community as well (and you don't need to wear the deli meat dress to do so). When I really dove into what it would take for me to start helping my own body – not just the medicine that was prescribed but really feeding my body what it needed to be as well as it could be - every single one of my friends thought I was going through a phase. Months later, after I dove head first into nutritional replenishing, hot yoga, meditation, and anything else I could find to help alleviate my own pain and inflammation, people would check in – "are you still doing that nutrition stuff?"

There were people who assumed that the weird stuff I was exploring was something I would come back from, but they didn't realize it was the weird stuff that was saving my life. A funny thing started to happen about a year in though - friends started asking for my advice. It was no longer "are you still doing that nutrition stuff?" but instead, "can you tell me about the energy work stuff you were talking about the other day?"

That full alignment with what it takes me to make sure I am well has turned into alignment for everything I am meant to be doing in my life. Embracing the weird, traveling down paths even when I did not personally know anyone else who would even try that particular path, is what has led me to more freedom to try out all sorts of things in my life. The courage it takes to be weird enough to try some sort of ancient healing method you think may work for you is the same courage it takes to be weird enough to throw all of your energy into a new business venture that you're not 100% sure about, but you really think has a chance of working.

People are watching. They're recognizing that, no matter what level of health they have, no matter what they're doing professionally, no matter where they are in life, they want to do better, feel better, and become better. What they once saw as weird, they're now realizing is the very thing they have to embrace to become the people they want to be. Your leading the way is hard, but it's helping your circle.

By being forced to go first, you're setting an example that many people never get to see. You're being the odd one out is bringing improvements to people's lives, even if they never muster up the courage to ask you directly about what you're doing. They're watching, and they're adapting these weird habits into their own lives as well, because at the end of the day, weird is best.

One of our modern world's favorite weirdos is Elon Musk, founder of PayPal, Tesla Motors, SpaceX, and SolarCity. He's like our very own representative from the X-Men – surely the only way he can be so weird and so smart is some kind of genetic mutation. But he is leading the way to our society working with our hands again, providing tangible solutions to problems like gas emissions, energy use, and space exploration. So many of our businesses and solutions these days are purely digital. The things that he creates are solving real-life problems that exist in our non-digital world, and that was his exact intent.

There is no arguing that Elon is truly unusual. In the 2015 biography written by Ashlee Vance, we not only learn about all of Elon's seemingly impossible schedules and ideas, but also of his highly eccentric parties. For Elon's 30th birthday party, he rented out a castle in England and played hide and seek from two to six o'clock in the morning with about twenty friends. Many of his parties end up being costume parties – for one, he showed up dressed as a knight and dueled a midget wearing a Darth Vader costume with his parasol (somehow, my question in all of this was why a knight would have a parasol). One of his big birthday blowouts had a Japanese steampunk theme; Elon dressed as a Samurai. He also famously said, before he remarried his previously ex-wife, that he wanted to find a girlfriend, but felt as though he needed to carve out more time. "How much time does a woman want a week?" he said. "Maybe ten hours? That's kind of the minimum? I don't know."

He is exacting. His mind is tortured by any kind of non-specific, or something that he doesn't deem as factual or logical. He is ridiculously particular. He is obsessed with all things actual technology and science, but also science fiction. One of his sons, Xavier, was specifically named after Professor X (see, he's definitely a member of the X-Men). But he also changed the way we use money online with PayPal, changed the landscape of the automobile with Tesla, rethought how we install and deliver solar panels on a large, usable scale with Solar City, and has drastically changed the prospect of space travel with Space X, where he has brought the cost of a single space mission down from $1 billion to $60 million in just a few short years. He is unapologetically, incredibly weird. By embracing that side of himself, he is changing the landscape and possible outcomes of our entire planet.

Your superpower, your own special thing that will help contribute toward making our planet a better one to live on, is your weirdness. Whether it developed by choice or by necessity, embracing it will not only change your own life but the lives of others. So let your freak flag fly, odd one. It is one of your many super powers, even if you got there by way of a really annoying thing that hasn't yet turned into a useful mutation. It's okay, we'll be inducted into the X-Men soon.

GRACE

When I was twelve years old, I got the amazing opportunity to travel to Taiwan and Hong Kong as a purposeful stowaway on a family business trip. It pulled me out of my seventh grade final exams, which I was not at all upset about, so that I could go and have the world be my teacher instead. For the record, my reasoning worked on every teacher except my geography and a world history teacher, which even then struck me as pretty ironic. I learned my fare share of geopolitical history; Taiwan and Hong Kong certainly has piles of it. But the thing I learned that took deepest root was a cultural lesson – that it is rude to turn down a gift.

My grandfather, who had been a prominent cardiovascular surgeon in New York City before he retired, had a friend who lived in Taipei. His friend, Mr. Jen, basically his Taiwanese counterpart, was also quite prominent in the same field, and also retired.

We met Mr. Jen early in our two week trip. He was tall, thin, and despite being well into his late 70s, had a way of death-gripping my 12-year-old self's arm as we walked through his apartment in Taipei to take in the view from his balcony. He seemed to take particular joy in making fun of me for how many dumplings I could down in a single sitting, but made sure to order more until I was completely full.

While I'm sure he mentioned many interesting and useful things over the course of our visit, the thing he imparted on me most was that in many Asian cultures, it was rude to turn down a gift of any kind. He wanted to make sure I was being culturally aware, and he said that this was the thing that he had a hard time forgiving from more western cultures. Other cultural differences could be accepted, but turning down a gift was a blatant affront to the gift-giver. It disrespected the time and thought they had put into a gift, no matter how little or much, and it took away the joy of giving a gift, which was often more than the joy of receiving one.

I had never thought of it that way before, but it made sense. While I wasn't exactly always great at picking out gifts (a particularly poor showing of my skills was the Christmas I ordered my entire family matching draft blockers for our doors - basically long tubes of horribly ugly fabric filled with sand), I took a lot of joy in researching what people might like. I loved wrapping presents creatively to try to bring a little whimsy into people's lives. It was an act of love, and I had never really thought about what it was to turn that gift away, even when it was in an effort to be polite or gracious.

In the American culture in particular, we don't always think of gift giving and accepting of it in this way. All throughout elementary and middle school history, we learn of the fiercely independent American explorers, forging their way through uncharted lands, supporting themselves in good times and bad. This is glossed over, of course. It says nothing to the communities set up, or the native American tribes people who helped along the way. This image of the lone ranger in the west is the ultimate symbol of the American way. We do this on our own. We don't need any help. We don't need gifts from others. We forge ahead.

In this way, I was a fiercely independent kid. I would have much rather failed hundreds of times over before asking for help. I wanted to know I could do things on my own. But that absolutely changed when I was diagnosed with type 1 diabetes at ten, even though I didn't realize the shift until much later. Of course I needed help giving myself shots. Of course I needed help from my medical team, my mom, my brother, my teacher, my school administrators, and my friends. But I think I almost saw it as something that could be sectioned off - of course I needed help with my disease. I was a kid, not a doctor. But that world stayed in its own little silo and I could still be fiercely independent with everything else.

Then along came Mr. Jen. I realized that people were giving me gifts in the form of their time and help, and that I was being rude and not honoring them by constantly turning them down.

So I started applying this lesson to my life, not just with my health, but with everything I did. An odd little transfer of energy was set up. By accepting others' gifts, be they time or help or actual tangible gifts, more gifts flowed my way. And only because of that, was I able to give more.

By college, it had taught me a supremely key lesson - to never be afraid to ask for help. People want to offer their knowledge, their time, their abilities. They want the opportunity to get involved, to rise to the occasion, to engage their own skills, to support others. It doesn't matter if you could have eventually gotten to it or figured out a way to do it on your own. By engaging the help of others, you have given the gift of community and mentorship. Others get to give you their gift of their skills and enthusiasm.

By living with chronic disease, you've already learned the skill of accepting gifts, even if you are the fiercely independent sort. At some point in time, you have leaned on a friend, a medical professional, a family member to help. And they wanted to - you leaning on them was your gift of trust and vulnerability. Have you started applying that superpower of asking for help to your other goals in life yet?

It's not a normal thing for humans these days to be good at doing, I can tell you that much. A quick Google search of 'business woman asking for help' will turn up thousands upon thousands of articles, all with just a slight variation on Why Do Women Find it So Hard To Ask for Help? It's certainly not a new concept – people have a hard time being vulnerable enough to ask for help. Particularly for women who identify with being overachievers and the type of woman who can do things on her own, asking for help can feel like you're letting yourself down. It's what makes me so particularly thankful that I have practice doing exactly what so many people struggle with. Our health has certainly caused massive issues in our life, there's no doubt about it. But sometimes, just sometimes, I actually get supremely thankful for what it's taught me, particularly when those lessons seem to be so far outside of what people typically do.

Sujan Patel, while writing for Forbes Magazine in December 2014, pointed out that there is an odd belief amongst young entrepreneurs in particular that to ask for help is weakness, even though asking for help is shown to lead to business growth and a more solid foundation for success. He goes on to state that asking for help not only boosts brand awareness (your ask just got your idea in front of more people), but is an excellent networking tool. By asking for help, you are finding like minded people, people who want to jump in, and people who are interested by what you do and therefore want to introduce you to other people who they think will be interested in what you do.

Love him or hate him, Jay Z is a master at asking for help. The guy collects mentors like no one else and, as one of the world's best selling artists who has 21 Grammys sitting at home (in addition to Beyonce's 18 – that has to be a sturdy set of shelves), is known as one of the most financially successful musical artists in the world, with a net worth of more than $450 million. He owns or co-owns clothing lines, clubs, record labels, video games, sports teams, restaurants, beauty lines, and advertising and sports agencies. He didn't start with all the skills to know how to do all of this – he asked people to help him learn. Not only has he sought mentors in fellow musicians like Russell Simmons and The Notorious B.I.G., but from athletes like Michael Jordan, media moguls like Oprah, business people like Bill Gates, and investors like Warren Buffett. When Jay Z identifies something he wants to do but doesn't know how, he asks.

This is something we learn, early and often, in our lives with our health. People aren't always going to chase you down to give you help, but by asking, you open the door for others to walk through.

I have a friend from high school whom I've watched do this particularly well. She lives in the Pacific Northwest with her husband and three young children and, over the past few years, has struggled with a myriad of health issues, often resulting in the need for bed rest, surgeries, and other painful procedures in an attempt to get her body healthy again. Meanwhile, she runs several online businesses, does periodic event planning work, writes for her personal blog, and wrangles her zoo of amazing but sometimes absolutely crazy kids.

When she knows she has an upcoming surgery or procedure, she does something simple but profoundly difficult for so many people – she puts out an ask for help on Facebook. She's got it down to a science. She creates a schedule for however long she knows she's going to need assistance and has her friends and family sign up for which days people can take the kids to or from school, sports practice, or camp. She asks people for a specific number of casseroles and family style dinners that can keep for a few days. She asks for people who can volunteer in shifts in her home to do the seemingly little things that would put a lot of strain on her body as it's recovering - things like straightening up and laundry. It's a planning marvel, but it's also a truly heart-warming thing to watch people jump in and sign up for tasks whenever her asks go up. Even 3,000 miles away, I find myself trying to figure out if I can order food to send her, just because my human drive to help kicks in.

Interestingly enough, her skill of asking is one I see her employ when she's well too. One of her online businesses is in network marketing, a business model specifically built on reaching out to people to ask if they'd like the services or product you're referring. All businesses require these specific asks. Even when you're offering services or products that can truly benefit someone's life, you're first asking for their time to listen. Mastering these asks for help – in the form of time, feedback, or even a purchase – is key to our success in anything and everything we do, so it's a great thing that we have so much practice.

My first job out of college was a communications position for the German American Chamber of Commerce in Atlanta. The organization's purpose was to help German companies who wanted to establish their business in the United States, and I was brought on to basically be the token American. It was my duty to make sure our communications aimed at the American market actually read well to an American audience. It was an interesting position and one that I stayed in for almost three years. Nearer to the end of my time there, I was able to hire an intern to help take on some of the work. We had gotten to the point where we were churning out a lot of content and events, and we needed more hands on deck to help out.

I got really lucky – the intern we hired, Morgan, was not only completely competent and a strong writer, but she was hilarious. A few months after she started, I got the offer to start contributing to our national business magazine. I was asked if I could write a monthly column aimed at helping German business people understand American cultural norms.

Let it be known, I am not a comedic writer or person in general. I get really awkward, really fast. My comedic timing is often cringeworthy, and far too many times I'm the only one thinking something is absolutely hilarious as people stare at me with a mixture of pity and annoyance. But I knew that, for this column to be good or reach people, it was going to have to use humor as a communication tool. Blandly listing a how-to was not going to be engaging.

On the other hand, my ego totally kicked in. A monthly column in a national magazine! It was a trade magazine and it's not like it had huge circulation, but at 24 it felt like a pretty big deal.

All the same, I sat with the offer for about an hour before I turned to Morgan and asked for her help. We ended up co-writing the column for almost a year, being able to bounce ideas off of each other, feed off of each other's writing style, and maniacally laugh at the cultural differences we kept stumbling across that were just downright strange. It was a well received project and by asking for help, not only were we able to actually put out something that was interesting and helpful, but the actual writing of it wasn't a chore. Getting help not only made the work more enjoyable, but made it better.

It then helped both of us with our careers. In our early 20s, we both had a major writing credit on our resumes, and it took nothing from either of us to have produced the work with someone rather than on our own.

Having to consistently ask for help with your health is exactly what teaches you to be vulnerable enough to ask for help in the rest of your life. Taking that skill learned in a difficult way and applying it to other aspects of your life is what helps you succeed. So many people struggle in silence with an increasingly overwhelming workload, or a problem that they just cannot figure out the answer to, thinking that asking someone for help is a weakness. It's a fantastic thing, then, that we have experienced things that help us know better. It is a superpower to know that asking for help is never a weakness, but is actually a strength. It is the putting aside of ego so that something better can happen as a result.

Not only that, but being transparent about what we need help with sets an amazing example for others. It gives them strength and takes away their fear. There is not a single person on this planet who doesn't have something they're struggling with, something that would truly benefit from someone else's help. But too many people are scared to admit it and scared that asking for help means they're not good or talented enough to figure it out on their own. In reality, it's just a life hack. Asking for help would help them get something done faster, more efficiently, and with less of a heavy lift. Not only that, but it would benefit the helper, teaching them a skill or just allowing them to feel useful and needed.

It's something my mom tells me every single time I call her asking for help. I'm in my late 20s, I feel like I should know the answer to more things than I do. But every time I start apologizing for having to reach out, she stops me. She reminds me that it's nice to feel needed, especially from your grown kid who's out in the world on her own and has been for ages.

In that way, it's a pretty cool gift, not only to ourselves but to others, that we know how to ask for help. It's just about applying it to all areas of our life instead of just our health. When we can take that superpower and harness it, we can turn it into an amazing level of success. The world functions on help from others. It's in our banding together that we create the greatest things.

SUPERPOWER #7
LEADERSHIP

think the heaviest burden of living with a chronic disease is knowing that it's forever. I know the type 1 diabetes community best, but I can imagine this is the age old adage across all chronic illnesses – a cure is less than ten years away. For the last eighteen years I've lived with T1D, a cure has always been ten years away. What was exciting to hear at first diagnosis has become a particularly exhausting joke.

I don't think it's a thought we allow ourselves to have often, but on the worst days, the days when you're in the most pain, or feeling the most tired, or the most nauseated, or whatever other barrage of symptoms you have to live with, it's a challenge to not sink into an incredibly dark place.

I've had these thoughts so maybe you've had them too - you've felt like this whole thing is never going to get better, so why try? Or maybe, in those particularly overwhelming moments, you've gotten thoroughly pissed off that this is never going away. Or maybe, instead of being pissed off, you've gotten deeply sad, to the point where you felt it in your core. It's beyond sadness. It's heartache.

It's a deep wish that you could have just been handed a normal life. You find yourself bargaining with whoever or whatever is out there making decisions – if this thing could just go away, you promise you'd be a million times better than you already are. And then you start thinking of all the things you would've done, could've done with this burden lifted. And you sink again. It is a heartbreaking cycle.

You have a good cry. You curl up with Netflix and a cup of tea, or Netflix and a bottle of wine (certain sinking episodes call for certain remedies). You hug your pet until he wriggles out of your arms in protest. You bury yourself in blankets. You go to sleep. You do anything you need to give yourself a well-deserved coddle so that when you wake up in the morning you can wash your face, down some coffee, put on your favorite outfit, and get to work.

It's why I have so much admiration for people who live with these illnesses looming in their lives. We tackle our dreams, just like we want to do, and we do it with an added weight on our shoulders that we are acutely aware is never leaving. We know this thing is going to be the constant interruption in our lives, and we find ways to accommodate it, fight through it, and even give it love by constantly thinking of it and finding the best ways to treat it. We remain undaunted. We remain powerful. If that's not a superpower, I truly don't know what is.

What gets particularly cool is when we take these hurdles and turn them into the drive to help others. It happens more often with people who go through challenging events than with anyone else I see. We know what it's like to carry this heavy weight and yet, instead of running forward to stay as ahead of it as possible, or just staying put and hiding in our safe space until everything is better, we reach back to help those struggling behind us.

Knowing what it's like to struggle makes us the best kind of leaders - the compassionate ones, the ones who lead with service. The ones who understand that the best feeling in the world is to turn around and lend a hand. It's actually incredibly self-serving, when you really think about it, but I think that's a great thing.

Combining self-care with leadership is a crafty little life-hack that I had the great fortune of learning pretty early. When I was 16 years old, I volunteered as a counselor at a camp for children and young adults with muscular dystrophy. My high school had a volunteer hours requirement - something like 100 hours for the four years you were in school - and me, being that I do absolutely nothing halfway (virtual high five if you're the same way), realized that I could knock out a large portion of these hours in one go at a sleepaway camp.

At this camp, I and one other teenage girl were paired up to help attend to the needs of a fellow young woman who could no longer eat, bathe, or dress herself. Together, we acted as her muscles, which had atrophied to a painful and debilitating point. It was hard work. We awoke several times a night to shift her in bed - without moving a few times over the course of the night she would wake up with excruciating cramps and joint pain. We woke up again before dawn to get ourselves ready before we lifted her out of her own bed into her motorized wheelchair and off to the showers, where we'd undress her, put her in her shower chair, and entertain her with our water fights while sudsing her down. We washed her face. We brushed her teeth. We got her dressed again.

We took her to the mess hall for breakfast, but would take turns scarfing down our own food so one of us could sit outside with her to help feed her. She didn't like eating with other people; she found it embarrassing. We stayed with her throughout the day, rolling along with her to different camp activities, trying to keep her spirits up as best we could. As tiring as we, 16 year olds who had never had this level of responsibility, were, we knew that it was absolutely nothing compared to the level of exhaustion that her constant pain put her in.

In the evenings, the washing of the face, brushing of the teeth, changing of the clothes routine started again. After one last stop to the bathroom, where we all sheepishly smiled at each other to try to ease our shared awkwardness, we would lift her into bed, adjust her legs and arms until she was comfortable, place her oxygen mask for her, then go off and get ourselves ready for bed too.

Whatever pats on the back I was getting for coming to volunteer time on my summer vacation, whatever acknowledgement I was getting for working so hard, I knew I was actually doing it all for a pretty selfish reason. At the end of that week, I was on a total high. I felt so valuable, so helpful. I liked how great giving myself that much to the camp made me feel. If I just felt exhausted at the end of it, like it had been a waste of my time, I probably wouldn't keep volunteering. In the end, helping others is actually a self-serving act.

It's not a bad thing. If we can help others and help ourselves at the same time, what's better? If, by knowing a sliver of what someone else may be going through, we can turn our compassion into a way to help, I can only see that as a damn good way to conduct ourselves as humans.

Throughout the week, my control of my T1D was the best it had been in a long time. Instead of thinking about it constantly, I was forced to put it behind someone else's needs. Every few days I would have an episode I needed to attend to, but otherwise it was all my camper, all the time. I think that having my own chronic disease made me aware to a small degree of what my charge was going through. Like her, my condition was never going to go away. But unlike her, I was still able to move through life with relative ease. While I had to take time outs often, I realized that I wasn't at all sidelined. I was just as capable of giving back and getting something valuable done as anyone else.

That's not to say that anyone ever gets to tell you that you have it worse or better than anyone else. I don't actually think that's helpful. At the end of the day, we all deal with frustration, with pain, with sadness, with heartbreak – these emotions are shared human experiences. This is what we're helping each other through. By experiencing these so often with our own health, we are uniquely equipped to help others tackle them too, no matter what is bringing them on. We all work within our abilities to give back what we can to our community.

And that's how we keep helping each other. It is only by realizing our own capabilities that we can continue to build each other up. We light each other's candles. We show each other the way.

I think we all know of a few prominent people in the world who do this well, and a few who point-blank don't. So many world leaders, business moguls, media stars seem to lack compassion in droves. I don't wish ill on anyone, but I do hope for a few people to get swift kicks of perspective sometimes.

On the other hand, the people we see who lead with compassion based on personal experience seem to emanate this sage-like glow. You can tell that they just know and it draws this certain charisma out of them. The charisma comes from truth, from alignment. It's something we possess too once we realize it.

Kris Carr, who we visited with in chapter three, has this glow. If you go check out a few of her YouTube videos, she has such an ethereal quality about her. It doesn't feel fake. It doesn't feel manufactured. It comes from a place of having been through the utter struggle and fear that she knows her audience may be going through, and truly wanting to wrap them up in this cocoon-like hug. When she sends out newsletters with the greeting, "Hey Sunflower," or "Hey Lovebug," it feels so genuine. Her experience of living with cancer for the past decade and what I can only imagine as the rollercoaster of emotions that has created, drives her to lead with love. And to give her just a few more pats on the back, remember that leading from such a genuine place of compassion has been particularly helpful for her career. Two of her books have been on the New York Times bestseller list and her service leadership has amassed her a huge following.

Sometimes it even seems like the people who go through the most give back in the most fearless ways. I had the amazing fortune to be friends with a guy named Guillaume when I was in college. Guillaume had deep brown skin, was tall and lanky, and had a particular love of dancing and cigarettes. He was from Africa but had grown up in Europe before coming to school in the states. He had a deep love for his people, for his home, and for supporting them however he could. He had figured out how to set up an importing business so that he could buy wares and items from home, ship them to America, sell them to high-ticket collectors, then send the money back home to those who needed it.

Specifically, Guillaume was from Rwanda. He was eight when the genocide happened. If you're not familiar, in 1994, in the midst of a civil war in the country, there was a genocide, a mass slaughter of the Tutsi people of Rwanda by the Hutu, who had a majority place in the government. It is unknown how many people died, but estimates are that between 500,000 and one million people were murdered in the matter of three months.

Guillaume's family was in a particularly difficult situation - his mother was Tutsi. His father was Hutu. What saved Guillaume's life was that his parents both had ties to important leadership who was able to smuggle their immediate family out of the country and north to Switzerland. He never told me how many people he knew died. I can only imagine it was most of them.

On a day when I was feeling particularly awful in college, Guillaume happened to wander by where I was sitting and ask me what was going on. I told him and explained that I was trying to figure out if I was going to go to work that day. I felt like calling out. I didn't feel like I could go deal with a bunch of rambunctious kids at the campus daycare where I worked.

He told me to go. He told me that the only way you can distract yourself is to keep going, to keep working, to find something to go take your mind off of it, even if only for a little while. I figured he knew best. I went.

It's what we all continue to do - despite not feeling our best; we keep going. We find a way, not only for ourselves but also for others. It is the best way to serve ourselves – to keep chasing what we've always wanted to chase. To keep going after whatever it is we would sprint toward if we found a magic potion to get rid of this thing tomorrow.

And here's the key thing – you are already a leader. You have already gone first in all of this. I'm willing to bet that you have friends who are struggling with chronic health issues as well, and they will watch your light. They may be trying to hide and go about life as if everything is normal, but they are going to keep an eye on how you live your truth.

It is time for you to go out into the world, with all of your superpowers, and be the entrepreneur, author, artist, business woman, actress, teacher, mentor, athlete, best woman blacksmith in the world, or whatever the hell else it is that you want to be.

You already have the super powers. This weird thing life handed you is teaching you everything you need to be great. You already know how to crush your goals. Now go make them happen.

"Happiness can be found even in the darkest of times,

if only one remembers to turn on the light."

DUMBLEDORE

THANK YOU

Thank you so much for reading Beyond Powerful! I'd love to hear what part of the book stuck with you most, or what you're going through that made you turn to this book. Please feel free to drop me a line at lala@lalajackson.com or find me anywhere on the internet – @heylalajackson.

Additionally, as a thank you for reading, please visit my website to check out a special, just for you, free video on the additional super power I know you have.

www.BeyondPowerfulBook.com

On occasion, I host personal and group workshops, speak, and lend my writing to other platforms. To learn more, book me as a speaker, or request a guest piece, visit www.lalajackson.com or email lala@lalajackson.com.

With ridiculous amounts of gratitude,

ABOUT THE AUTHOR

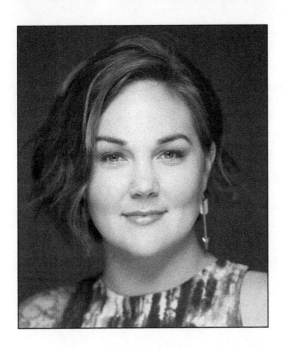

L ala Jackson has been navigating the world of being an over-achieving go-getter who lives with chronic disease since she was 10 years old and diagnosed with the autoimmune disease type 1 diabetes. She is a writer, speaker, and advocate for fellow young people living with invisible illness.

Lala lives in Brooklyn and works for a non-profit whose mission is to cure type 1 diabetes. She loves traveling to literally anywhere with a swim-able beach, whipping up a paleo concoction, attempting to not fall over in yoga, throwing paint on a canvas, or flat out sleeping. Because knowing when to rest is everything.

She grew up between Hawaii and Washington State, graduated from the University of Miami in Florida with a communications degree, has a heart for all things multicultural, and is obsessed with recognizing all of us are beyond powerful – because chasing dreams while living with chronic disease is no small task. She's also a Gryffindor.

For more information visit:
lalajackson.com

For speaking and writing inquiries,
or for any other questions, email:
lala@lalajackson.com

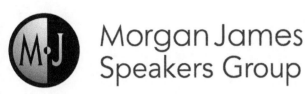

Morgan James
Speakers Group

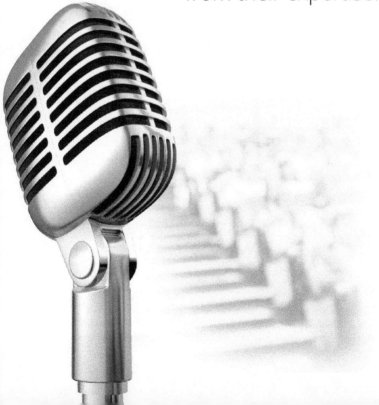

www.TheMorganJamesSpeakersGroup.com

We connect Morgan James published
authors with live and online events
and audiences whom will benefit
from their expertise.